PRINCIPLES AND PRACTICE OF KINTAPE

A EXPLORATION OF HOW KINTAPE CAN EFFECT THE HUMAN BODY

HAN SHIBING

TABLE OF CONTENTS

Chapter I: Introduction to Kintape...1
    Part I: What Is Kintape?.....................................1
    Part II: Types of Kintape 4
    Part III: Kintape Construction Materials....................9
    Part IV: Benefits of Kintape............................11
Chapter II: Principle of Kintape 17
    Part I: An Origin - Bionics 17
    Part II: Six Functional Principles......................28
    Part III: Principles & Interrelation of Product Parameters...........40
Chapter III: Taping Methods................................47
    Part I: Basic Knowledge For Structures of Human Body.............47
    Part II: Precautions For Operation and Method.........................51
Chapter IV: Common Adverse Reactions and Causes 75
Chapter V: Practical Taping Methods For Various Body Parts..........83

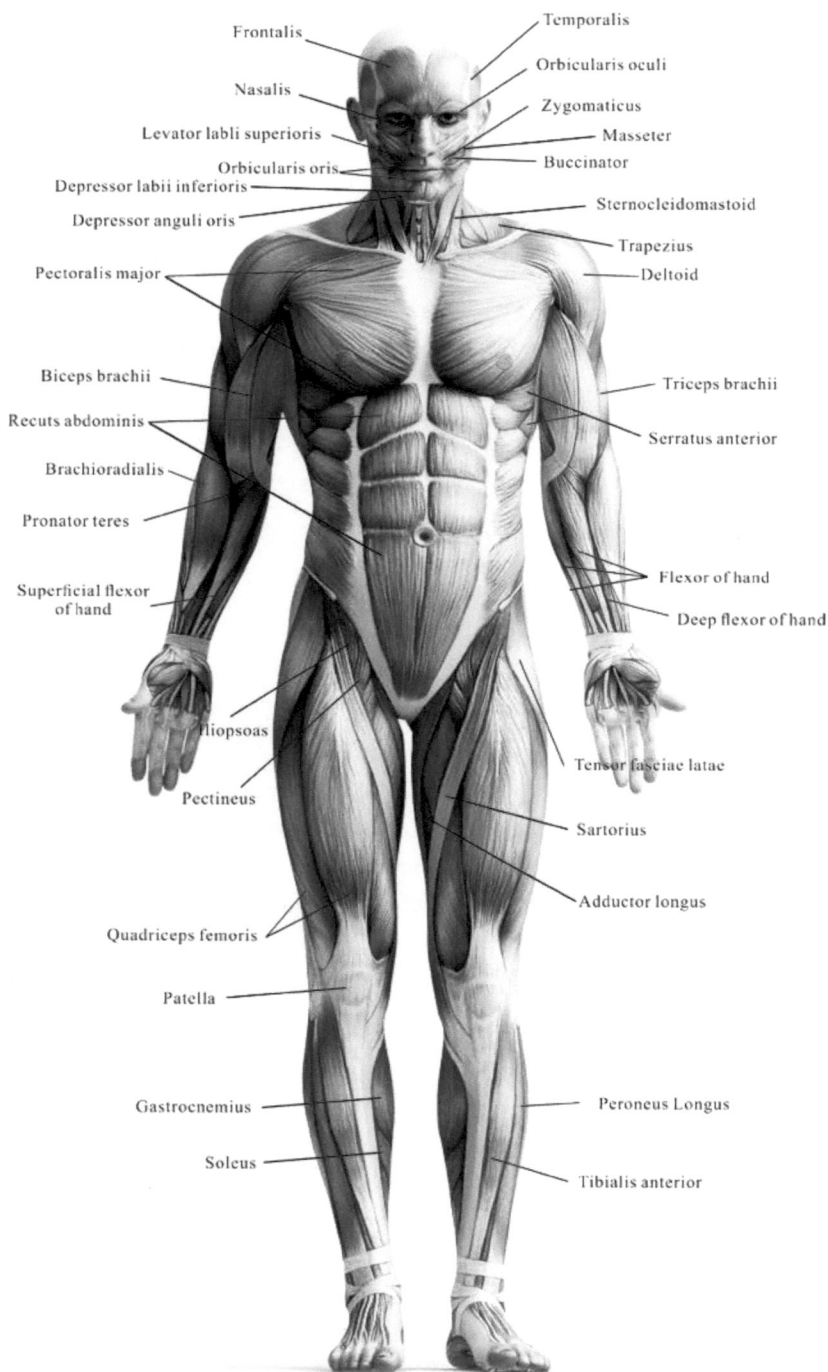

Frontalis

Temporalis

Orbicularis oculi

Nasalis

Zygomaticus

Levator labli superioris

Masseter

Orbicularis oris

Buccinator

Depressor labii inferioris

Depressor anguli oris

Sternocleidomastoid

Trapezius

Pectoralis major

Deltoid

Biceps brachii

Triceps brachii

Recuts abdominis

Serratus anterior

Brachioradialis

Pronator teres

Superficial flexor
of hand

Flexor of hand

Deep flexor of hand

Iliopsoas

Pectineus

Tensor fasciae latae

Sartorius

Adductor longus

Quadriceps femoris

Patella

Gastrocnemius

Peroneus Longus

Soleus

Tibialis anterior

Diagram of Human Frontal Muscles

Occipitalis
(back the scalp)

Trapezius

Spine of scapula

Deltoid

Infraspinatus

Teres Minor

Latissimus dorsi

Teres Minor

Musculus triceps brachii

Extensor carpi radialis longus

Lumbodoral fascia

Extensor digitorum
communis

Flexor and Extensor

Iliac crest

Gluteus Med

Gluteus maximus

Biceps femoris

Semitendinosus

Semimembranosus

Gastrocnemius

Achilles tendon

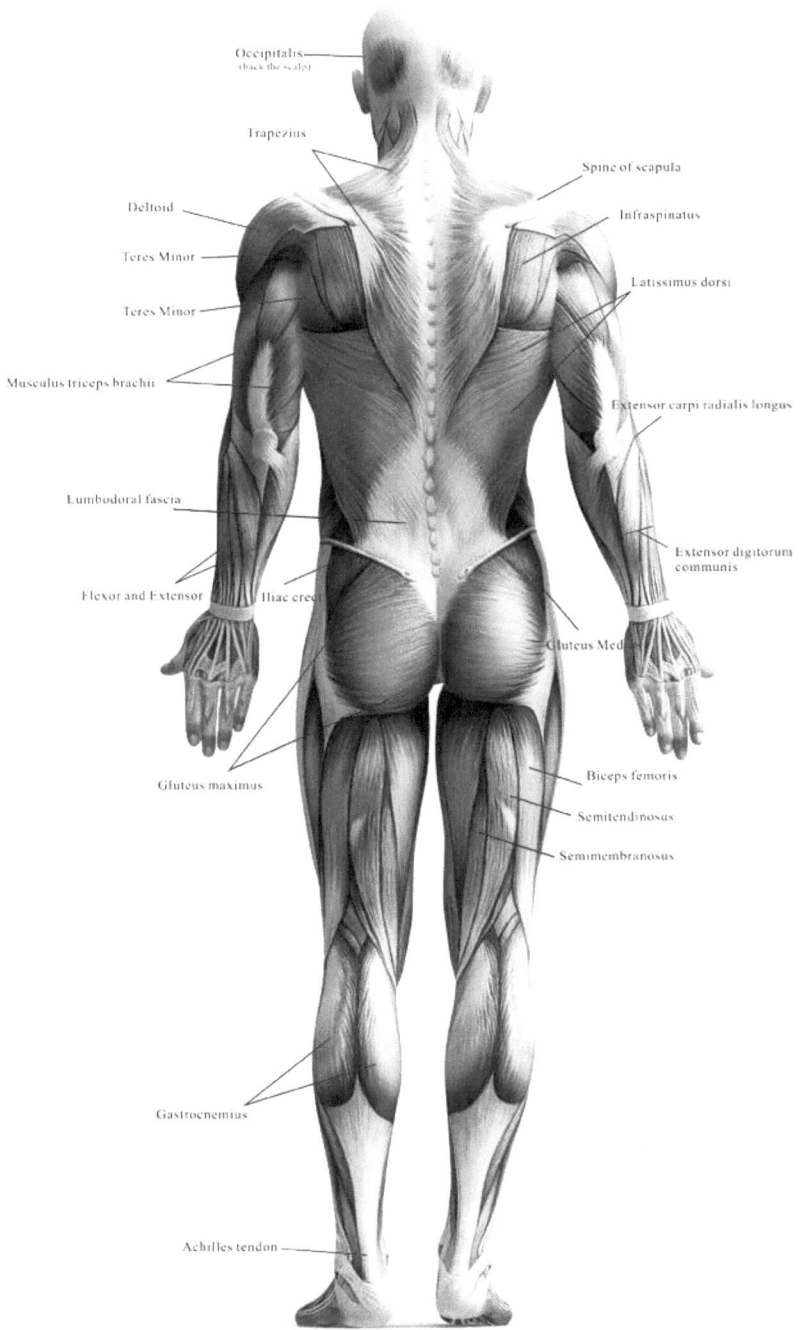

Diagram of Human Rear Muscles

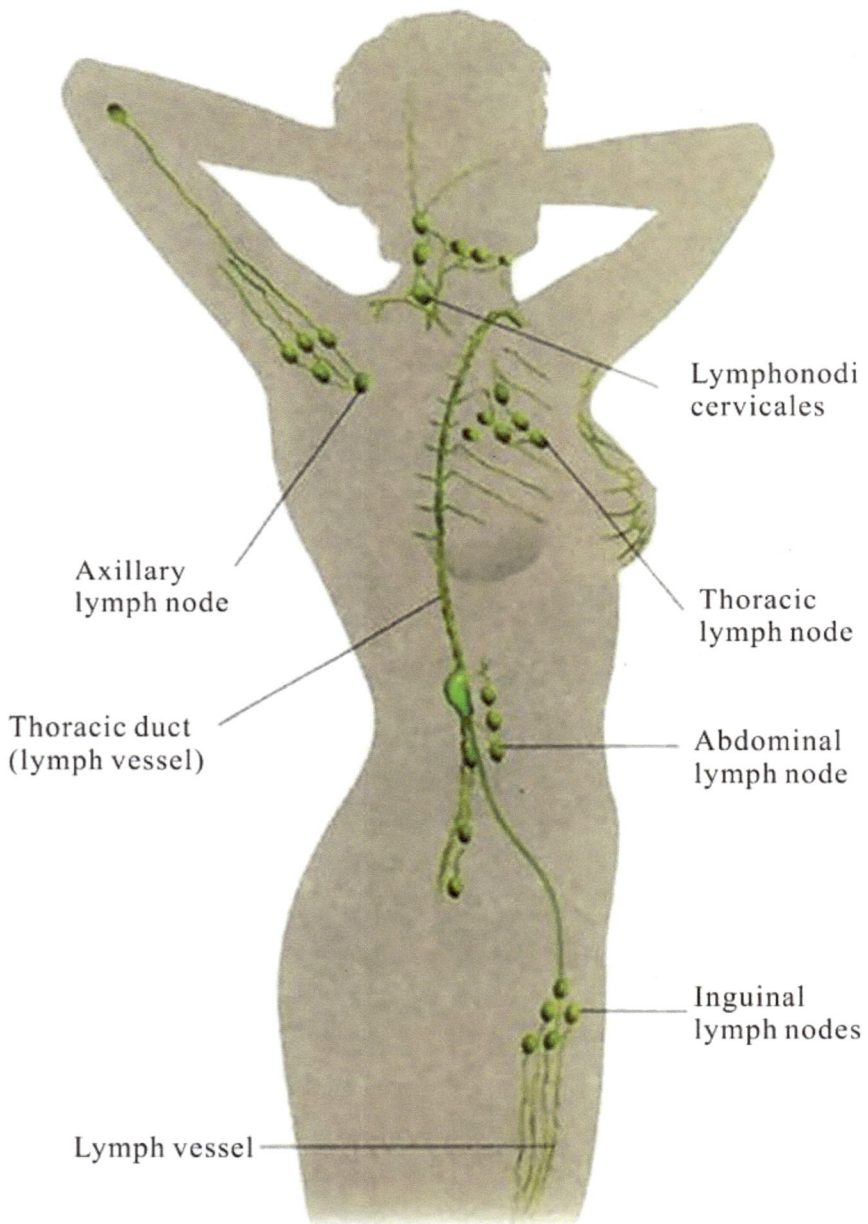

Lymphonodi
cervicales

Axillary
lymph node

Thoracic
lymph node

Thoracic duct
(lymph vessel)

Abdominal
lymph node

Inguinal
lymph nodes

Lymph vessel

Diagram of Human Lymphatic System

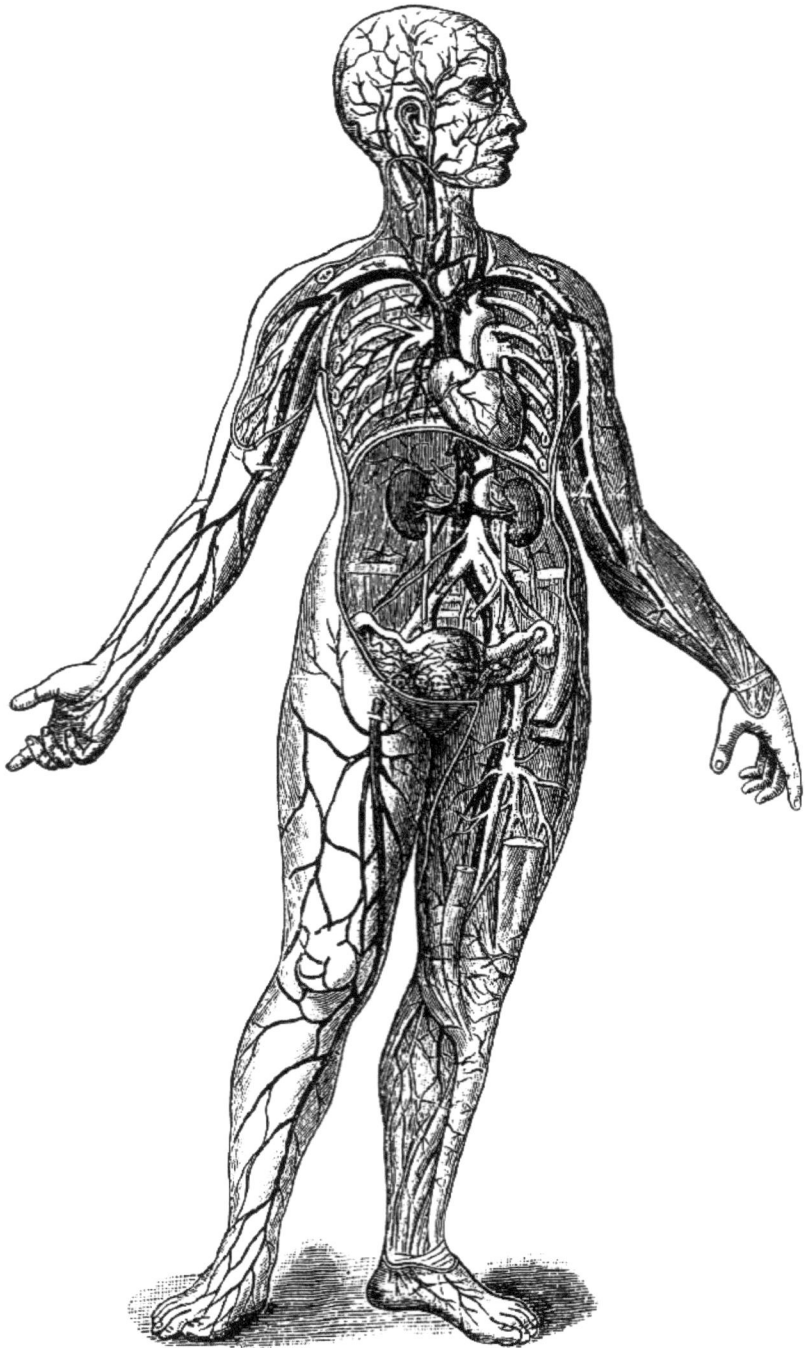

Diagram of Human Blood Vessels

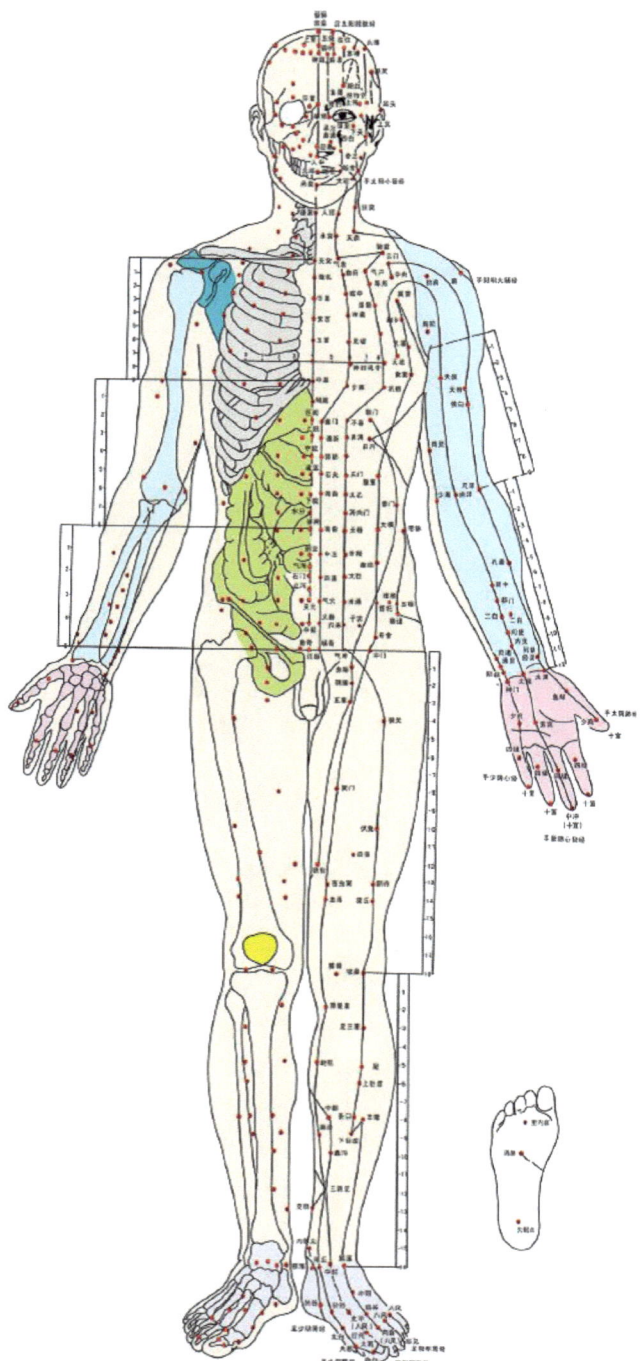

Diagram of Human Frontal Acupoints

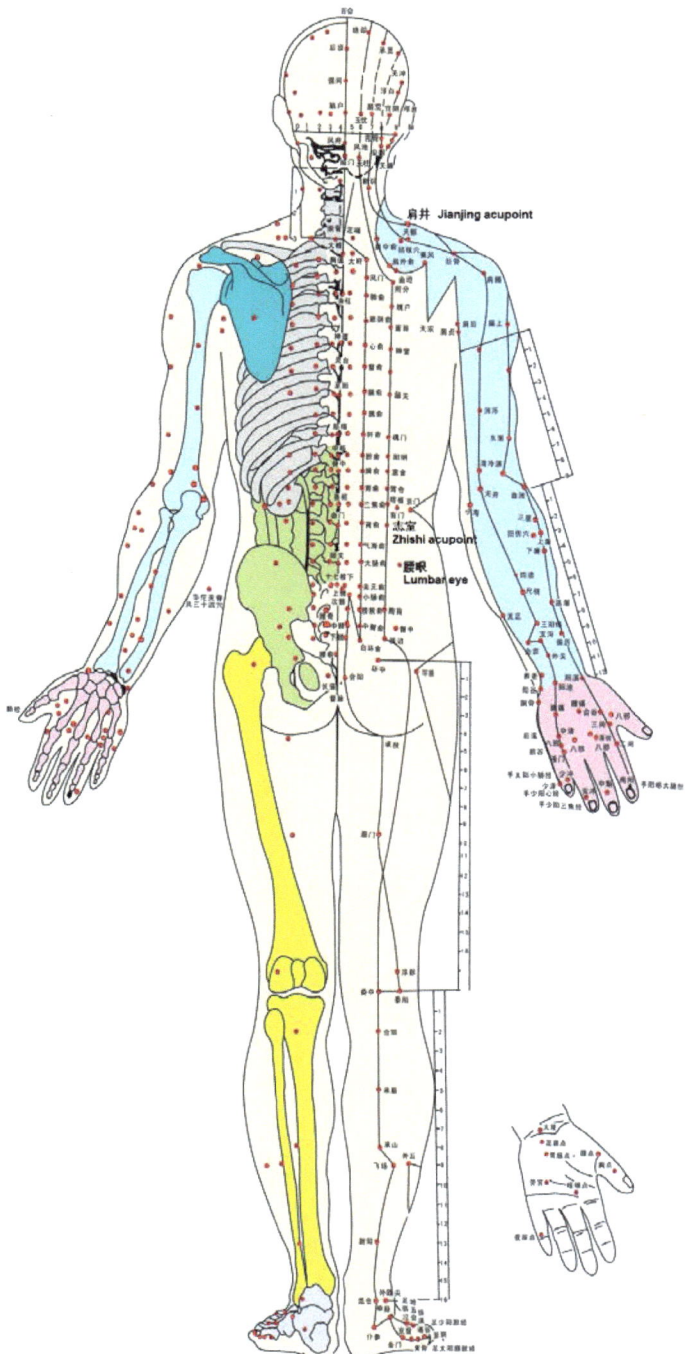

肩井 Jianjing acupoint

志室 Zhishi acupoint

腰眼 Lumbar eye

Diagram of Human Rear Acupoints

CHAPTER I: INTRODUCTION TO KINTAPE

PART I:
WHAT IS KINTAPE

Kintape, also known as , is a kind of tape that is beneficial to the human body through its various interactions with human organizational structures. Positive results stem from certain usage techniques, operation specifications, and physical methods.

We may conclude from its name that first of all, kintape is a kind of tape. It is, in fact, a cloth material that can be applied onto human skin by certain adhesion programs or applications. In most applications, glue that is harmless to the human body or with minor side effects where—after comprehensive consideration and testing—the beneficial effects are determined to be far greater than the harmful, shall be selected. Of course, there are still other countless feasible programs regarding the principle as well as methods, e.g. adsorption, acetabulum just like those of geckos, and other adhesion programs. With the development of science and technology, we will undoubtedly be discovering and adopting additional adhesion programs and applications.

The application of the tape must be beneficial to the human body. In cases where there are some harmful effects, the beneficial effects must be far greater than its harmful ones. This is a point that can be easily understood: if no obvious benefit is found or its harmful effects are greater than its beneficial ones, the product shall not be applied to the human body. For example, if glue with serious irritability effects on the human body is selected, although it may result in positive changes to the human body, serious irritability and even negative effects (e.g. sores or festering wounds) will also result. Thus, the product cannot be applied to the human body as qualified kintape. Moreover, it cannot even be categorized as kintape.

Kintape adopts physical methods, which are different from chemical and biological methods, to act on the human body. Particular attention should be paid to this because physical methods will achieve specific functions by changing the capabilities of the products or forming corresponding interactions with certain operational systems of the human body through its external physique changes. Since they are physique changes, the range of variation is infinite. To achieve beneficial effects, however, the range of variation must be limited, rather than extended infinitely or beyond the bearable range of the human body. For example, if a portion of an arm will get swollen and painful when it is struck, we may massage it gently to relieve the pain. It is a physical method. However, if we impose huge force—exceeding the bearable pressure range of the human body—acute pain and even additional injuries may be caused. This principle is fully applicable to kintape products. For kintape products, using physical methods is the greatest feature in their application, i.e. physical therapy.

During the application of the product, interactions must be formed between the kintape and one or more function(s) of the human body. The range of "interactions" here is relatively complex, and does not refer solely to the reactions in our skin or muscles that will result after kintape is applied. This is because the human body's systems themselves are relatively complex, and we are continuously learning about the operational systems of the body, understanding that no one solution will work for every person, disease, or injury. There are various internal and external systems, as well as joint points. For example, although the blood has its unique operational system, intersections with the lymphatic system may also be found. When we take one of the interactions into consideration, another unneeded interaction may be created.

Once kintape is applied to the human body surface, the affected range may not only be limited to the skin or muscles onto which it is applied, but also include blood vessels and nerves, etc. In addition, everyone has their own individual differences, requiring the operator of the kintape to give consideration to these differences to the furthest extent possible, in order to make every comprehensive interaction develop towards a beneficial direction and avoid negative interactions with the human body. After all, the understanding of science for the human body is still on the path of improvement and discovery.

We have talked about physical methods and their interactions with the human body. Therefore, it is easy for us to recognize that to achieve the most beneficial results within the ability of the operators, there must be an operation technique or specification. This operation specification, regardless of the impact of kintape products on the human body, may not be ideal. It must minimize the negative effects within the range of understanding, and different understandings and operation techniques may occur since effects and ranges of diseases and injuries vary. Furthermore, additional operation techniques and specifications may result from different medical systems and training programs. No matter which method is selected, though, we shall always consider problems from the perspective of the negative to avoid negative effects based on our existing knowledge.

Common forms of kintape are as follows:

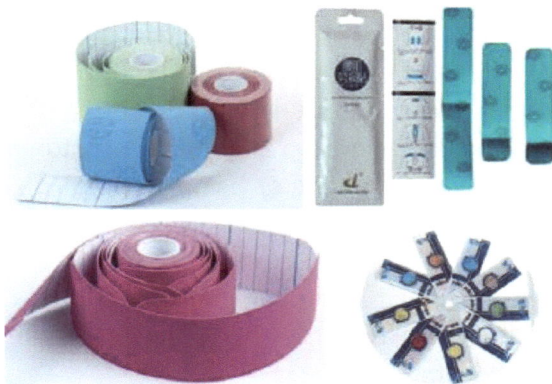

PART II:
TYPES OF KINTAPE

A simple conclusion may be drawn, based on its definition and constituents, that all tape products applied onto and beneficial to the human body can be called kintape. In a broad sense, this conclusion, which may cover thousands of products, is certainly correct. The kintape we discuss in this book, however, is designed as a specific series of products with the following external characteristics:

1. The products are of intrinsically elastic force. The "elastic force" here refers to warp-wise elastic force, which means the tape must have lengthwise elastic force, regardless of whether the products have widthwise (crosswise) elastic force. The most basic requirement for the elastic force is that one should feel obvious lengthwise extension when the tape is pulled by hand.
2. They have a high resilience ratio, which means that after being pulled, the tape must return to its original or nearly original length immediately. The "immediately" here can be understood or specified thusly: after the external force is removed, the time for spring back and removal of external force are seamlessly connected and synchronically completed. This is in contrast to elongation ratio, where the tape may be extended (such as lengthened) without returning to its original or nearly original length after the external force is removed, or slow elastic force, where the article is returned to its original or nearly original length after the external force is removed, but the whole process cannot be completed immediately.
3. High viscosity. For kintape products, a main feature that makes them different from many tape or bandage products is how they are used. Kintape products are applied onto the surface of the human body, while many other products are circumvoluted around the surface of the human body to achieve the effects required. High viscosity, therefore, becomes an important characteristic of kintape products.

4. It must have certain effects with a certain theoretical basis. Any one product may be effective for people of a certain type of physique, but may not necessarily be effective for people of other physiques. Therefore, the effect assessment is generally certified by two means: clinical results and the theoretical basis. Currently, for the certification of clinical results, operating methods and usage principles have not been unified, and technical parameters provided by manufacturers and the parameters of brand products are diverse. Even with the scientific developments and advancements in understanding the human body, explanations made by various medical systems for the interactions in and of the human body are not the same. Even the features of various products provided by the same manufacturers are different. Thus, we still cannot obtain completely consistent results for the whole product series of kintape, or effective, standard data recognized by all parties. The product series of kintape mentioned above, therefore, must have its own completely effective results that are based on existing scientific recognition and that can be theoretically derived.

Such a specific series of kintape products must have the several unique features mentioned above. Among specific products having the above several features, we can make the following classifications:

1. RAW MATERIALS:
   a. All cotton and spandex. The warp yarn is made of all cotton and spandex filament, which is used to produce elastic force, while the weft yarn is made of all cotton;
   b. All cotton and latex thread. The warp yarn is made of all cotton and latex thread, which is used to produce elastic force, while the weft yarn is made of all cotton;
   c. Staple fiber, or rayon and spandex;
   d. Staple fiber, or rayon and elastic spandex filament;
   e. Elastic nylon—generally made of PA66;
   f. Elasticity-enhanced polyester silk or other elasticity-enhanced products;
   g. Other materials.

2. CONSTRUCTION METHODS:
   a. Woven fabrics, which refer to fabrics formed by interweaving the warp and weft yarns of the material;
   b. Knitted fabrics, which refer to fabrics that are formed by the knitting of materials, resulting in a material more flexible than woven fabric;
   c. Other construction methods including non-fabric (e.g. elastic non-woven fabrics), three-dimensional weaving, leno weaving, etc.

3. WEAVING STRUCTURES:
   a. Plain weave, which refers to fabrics formed by interweaving weft and warp yarn up and down;
   b. Leno weave, which refers to fabrics formed by two warp yarns twisted around the weft yarns. Also known as Gauze weave or Cross weave;
   c. Rip weave (including warp rip and weft rip), which refers to fabrics formed by two, three, or more parallel warp or weft yarns as one in a weaving circulation;
   d. Other weave, which refers to weave with variability, e.g. twill and satin weaves.

4. THE DIRECTION OF ELASTIC FORCE:
   a. Warp-wise elastic kintape, which refers to kintape products with warp-wise elastic force only;
   b. Warp and broad-wise elastic kintape, which refers to products with both warp and broad-wise elastic forces;
   c. Omnidirectional elastic kintape, which refers to kintape with elastic forces in all directions. This product is mainly manufactured by knit methods.

5. CATEGORIES OF GLUE. SINCE THERE ARE NUMEROUS TYPES OF GLUE, SOME SPECIALIZED, WE WILL ONLY CATEGORIZE GLUES COMMONLY USED WITH KINTAPE:
   a. Medical acrylic acid glue, which is also called acrylic glue. It is the main glue applied to kintape products at present. All products mentioned hereinafter refer to kintape with glue of this type;

b. Kintape with medical hot melt glue, which is being eliminated gradually but still used by some manufacturers. It is mainly applied in the sports field;

c. Zinc oxide glue. It is listed separately as the gluing mode is different. When applying zinc oxide glue, various medical components can be added. One characteristic of zinc oxide is that it may shrink the skin, so pain can be reduced when peeling off kintape;

d. Hot melt zinc oxide glue, i.e. to add proportional zinc oxide to hot melt glue;

e. Various ingredients, such as nano gold, titanium, negative ion powder, mineral substances, and ion copper, are added to acrylic acid glue to strengthen one or more of the functions of kintape products.

6. FORMS OF GLUE SURFACES:

a. Vertical bar glue, i.e. the glue surfaces are in forms of vertical bars; in this circumstance, sometimes the glue surfaces may be in interrupted form for ventilation. However, if they are cut into small rolls rather than onto the glue surfaces, deckle edges will occur. Due to this disadvantage, few products of this type can be found now;

b. S ripple glue, surfaces that are in end-to-end arrangement on the tapes in "S" forms. This is the mainstream product as well as the product discussed in this book;

c. Horizontal bar glue, i.e. glue surfaces are in a side-to-side arrangement on the tapes in forms of horizontal bars. In this circumstance, sometimes the glue surfaces may be in interrupted forms. This was the glue surface adopted for kintape when it was first released, and is the patented technology of a Japanese company;

d. Slanted bar glue surfaces, i.e. glue surfaces regularly arranged with fabrics in certain angles;

e. Special figures including regular geometric shapes (such as rhombus and spots) or combinations of the glue shapes above.

The product discussed in this book is elastic kintape of plain woven fabric and medical acrylic acid S ripple glue. For convenience, it is hereinafter referred to as kintape. Products in other categories will not be described in this book as the principles do not apply.

Common forms of kintapes are as follows:

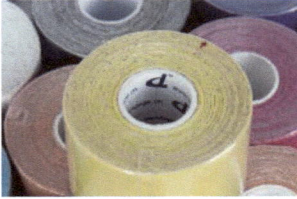

All Cotton

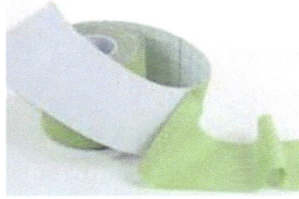

Rayon

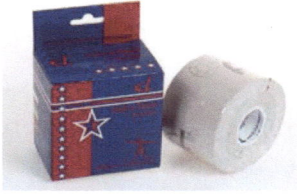

Four-way Spandex

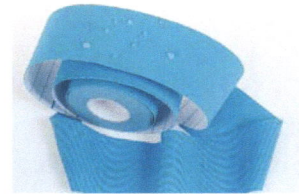

Glue Surface

PART III:
KINTAPE CONSTRUCTION MATERIALS

For products mentioned in this book, the main ingredient of warp yarns refers to cotton fiber, and the weft yarns are 100% cotton. Kintape made of other ingredients will not be mentioned.

Kintape is also called all-cotton kintape. In fact, this name is not totally accurate as the material construction of kintape products can be divided into several parts:

I. INGREDIENTS OF FABRICS

Since warp yarns are of elastic force, a certain proportion of spandex filament is contained in the warp yarns of products. Depending on the thickness and density of the yarns (which may be changed by yarn twist), the thickness of spandex filament, and the total weight of yarns per unit area, the proportion of the cotton and spandex of each brand is different. Generally, the proportion is approximately: cotton, 97% - 98%; spandex filament, 2% - 3%. Thus, it is not a proper description that the product consists of 100% cotton. The weight of fabrics in kintape is about 50% of the final product.

II. PROPORTION OF GLUE

The glue is an important component of kintape. The gluing rates of products of each brand are different. Of the total weight of kintape, on average, the weight of glue accounts for about 20% (based on dry glue of 70 g).

Medical acrylic acid glue (acrylic glue) is commonly applied as it has the most suitable initial and holding viscosities with extremely low irritability for the human body at present. The commonly-used curing rate is about 50% (50% glue + 50% solvent). Although ingredients adopted by each manufacturer vary, the solvent should be completely volatilized in the manufacturing process or it may cause anaphylaxis or another allergic reaction. The most commonly used solvent is acetic ether.

III. RELEASE PAPER

The thickness of the release paper adopted by commonly used kintape is about 0.12 mm (kintape requiring die cutting is thicker) with silicone oil and wax covering one side. Its gram weight is about 100 g/m^2 (for the kintape requiring die cutting, 120 g/m^2). Thus, the release paper of regular kintape accounts for about 30% of the whole kintape product.

The structural scale diagram for kintape is as follows:

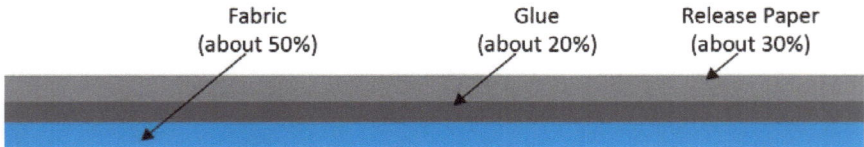

Fabric
(about 50%)

Glue
(about 20%)

Release Paper
(about 30%)

PART IV:
BENEFITS OF KINTAPE

Kintape is designed to change functions of the human body through physical methods. However, what improvements can be brought to the human body by kintape? What is the application scope of kintape?

1. INFLUENCE ON SKIN

Kintape is directly applied onto the skin surface, thus a direct influence on skin will be created, which has two possibilities. On the one hand, it may be beneficial to the skin; for example, it may remove subcutaneous melanin or lower the speed of subcutaneous melanin formation, accelerate subcutaneous blood circulation, and broaden subcutaneous space. On the other hand, it may cause a negative reaction to the skin, including skin surface injuries, red dots on the skin surface, and strong gargalesthesia. The main reason for these reactions is that the product will make the skin move toward one direction. When the movement exceeds the bearable range of the skin, injuries may be caused, just like damages and discomfort will be caused if we tighten our skin by hand for a long time. In addition, direct injuries can also be caused by glue, i.e. damages can result from peeling off the kintape incorrectly, as well as the over-viscosity of glue as it is applied onto the skin.

The injury as shown in the fig. below can be prevented when glue is applied onto the skin. See Chapter III, Part II for the proper methods of applying kintape.

Skin is crinkled under the glue and damages will result

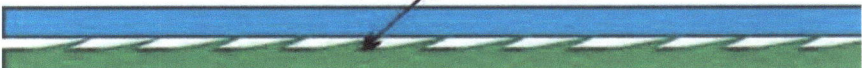

2. INFLUENCE ON MUSCLES

Though Kintape is applied to the skin, it can also be considered as applied onto muscles, leading to an obvious influence on muscles. This is the point to which many operators or researchers pay the most attention. Different effects will be caused depending on if the direction of applied elastic force is the same or opposite the direction of muscular force. Strong beneficial effects will be created by when kintape is applied correctly, and with knowledge of the functions of the muscles and how they respond to kintape. Of course, poor understanding of muscles, the basic principle of this product, or the use of unqualified products may result in unexpected or even opposite results.

3. INFLUENCE ON NERVOUS SYSTEM

The nerve conduction is influenced by the direction of applied force. Additionally, the product contains powerful functionality, which may accelerate the break over of neurons.

4. INFLUENCE ON BLOOD

The flow guidance function of the product as well as its principle and methods will be discussed in detail in Chapter II. Since the blood, which is of certain directivity, is flowing and the product has the function of guide the flow through proper application, the product is able to control the flow rate and/or direction of blood.

5. FUNCTIONS TO LYMPH AND LYMPH GLANDS

The lymph can be changed by adjusting the flow rate or direction of the liquid in interstitial fluid. This is the same as the principle of adjusting the flow rate or direction of blood. It can either introduce the lymph in lymph glands to inflammation points or collect the lymph together to provide concentrated diminishing inflammation.

6. FUNCTIONS TO SKELETON

The product can fix skeletons suffering from transformation or functional changes. It can put bones in place or reduce pain by providing support relying on the its physical transformability and fastening capacity. The same product can be applied to convey the different abilities of elastic recovery and anti-acting force in different parts with different stretch rates, depending on how and where it is used. In addition, different strength points will be created when applied onto different parts of the body with different strengths, and differences in moments of force will be generated, i.e. it may fix the skeleton, put it in place, or provide support for it.

7. OTHER FUNCTIONS

Functions and applications such as fixing, binding, pressing, shape rectifying, truncation, and subcutaneous space opening have been discovered, and additional functions will continue to be invented and explored with the summation and accumulation of the experiences of users, as well as the upgrades and changes made to the product and our understanding of its functions.

The application scope discussed above is only from the perspective of the different systems constituting the human body. From the perspective of the product itself, it is only a classification based on its physical characteristics. In practical application, however, we always deal with various kinds of discomfort in the human body, the causes of which differ from one case to another. How can we tell, then, which diseases and injuries can be dealt with by this product and which cannot?

The functions of kintape are most often achieved through physical therapy. Generally speaking, all injuries that can be dealt with by this product are caused by or result in non-bacterial inflammation. It shall be noted that the product can also deal with bacterial inflammation but since the characteristics of bacteria cannot be identified clearly, the diminishment of bacterial inflammation shall be prohibited to avoid serious adverse reactions.

Inflammation in the human body can be divided into bacterial and non-bacterial inflammation. Bacterial inflammation refers to injuries to the human body resulting from the generation, reproduction, and growth of bacterial organisms. For example, viral influenza is caused by a virus, to which the product is not effective; moreover, the product cannot deal with the inflammation, festering, and ulceration of wounds caused by bacterial infections. For non-bacterial inflammation or pain, however, the correct use of suitable products will reduce the discomfort of the human body. For example, the removal of acidic materials resulting from unbearable external force and the elimination or reduction of the inflammation accumulated by long-term strains.

In regards to telling a bacterial inflammation from a non-bacterial one, this method below can be adopted: bacterial inflammation has the ability of self-replication. It will conduct self-replication and reproduction under any circumstances as long as external conditions remain, and chemical or biological methods are always needed to eliminate it effectively. For non-bacterial inflammation, however, it only has the ability of continuous accumulation rather than self-replication, but a lack or reduction of the self-repairing capability of the human body may make it constantly accumulate at injured points and increase the extent of damage.

In addition, the application scope of this product can also be categorized based on differences in the sensations of the human body. Excluding the causes of bacterial inflammation, the sensations of the human body mainly include:

1. DOTTED PAIN
   This refers to independent pain on a point of the human body's surface or muscles that is not related to adjacent muscles or skin.

2. NERVOUS TENSION
   Generally, this refers to a sense of tension in veins or muscles. For example, the rear and lateral side of the thigh, even to the leg (shank) and foot for some individuals with serious symptoms; spasms are barely seen in most parts (e.g. the back of the knee).

3. MUSCLE WEAKNESS
   This generally results from the strain of muscles caused by repetition of the same action over a long time; a sense of weakness will arise. For example, weakness of the waist/lower back suggests straining of the lumbar muscles.

4. PAIN
   Generally, pain will occur after the muscles, skeleton, or ligaments are injured.

5. MUSCLE STIFFNESS
   This is generally caused by the reduction or loss of the blood flow of muscles, resulting from a long-term static or relatively immobile state of the blood in muscles, usually by the muscles being kept in one posture or state for extended periods. This will ultimately result in the blood circulation becoming blocked in muscles. In addition, it can sometimes arise from unbearable strength imposed on the muscles, or injuries of the nervous system in muscles, which will result in movement functional disorder.

6. SORENESS
   This is mainly caused by hyperkinesis, i.e. muscle spasms or cramps. Exercises exceeding the bearable range of muscles will result in muscle hypoxia, which will lead to acid build up.

7. NUMBNESS
   This is mainly caused by a nervous breakpoint or insufficient blood supply.

8. SWELLING
   The break of blood capillaries may result in poor local blood flow.

9. SPECIFIC UNCONTROLLED MUSCLES
   They mainly result from a damaged nerve conduction system, as well as the excessive strain of muscles.

10. OTHER SYMPTOMS

Under most cases, a complex rather than single symptom will occur if the balance of the human body is broken. Those symptoms (e.g. headaches after drinking and unexplainable pain in the back) or their causes also fall within the application scope of kintape.

CHAPTER II: PRINCIPLE OF KINTAPE

PART I:
AN ORIGIN – BIONICS

I. SURFACE FORMS OF KINTAPE

Kintape consists of three parts: the fabric, the glue, and the release paper. The glue surface shown below will appear after the release paper is peeled off.

How can a glue surface of this kind make such powerful changes to the human body? What if we replace it with other types of glue surfaces? A most fundamental design aesthetic, which is sometimes ignored by manufacturers, researchers, and operators, shall be considered to this end. Generally, this ability can be explained from the perspective of the waves of the glue surfaces, however it is insufficient in clarifying the reason functions can be introduced by waves or other forms.

Furthermore, many training institutions or manufacturers may certify the effect of a product through the senses of the human body or results in form changes after application; the form changes of subcutaneous fascia organizations before and after the application of kintape are usually taken as the contrastive case. Although this is correct, the reason why waves or other specific forms are adopted by glue surfaces cannot be clarified with those results, so the explanation is incomplete. It is similar to explaining the nutrients in food by the sense that someone is full; having a full stomach is not equal to the food containing needed nutrients.

Thus, we shall clarify the reason why glue surfaces in the form of waves and other kinds are adopted. Other shapes of glue surfaces can be designed, more effective products can be manufactured, and effective guidance can be introduced to our practical operation rules only if the theoretical problem is solved.

Before explaining this fundamental principle, I'd like to provide you a quick review to a most fundamental structure of the human body.

STRUCTURE OF VEINS IN THE HUMAN BODY

If we take the heart as the starting point of blood circulation, we shall use it as the terminal point, too. As the heart beats, the blood flows to the arms and legs through arteries, and returns to the heart through veins after the interchange of materials. This is how a complete circulatory system is formed. While the principle is easy to understand, it becomes more complex once an additional influence is added: the earth's gravity.

When we stand on the ground, the heart is located at the position a little above the center of the human body. The strong pressure resulted from heartbeats is definitely able to push the blood into the top of our heads, while the blood can flow down even easier, as the earth's gravity alone is sufficient to draw the blood back into our toes regardless of other factors. The problem, however, occurs in the later stage: when the blood returns to the heart through the veins, the pressure delivered by the heart is not sufficient to draw the blood from the toes back to the heart in opposition to the earth's gravity. In addition, the heart beats through contracting and expanding. When the heart is contracting, the pressure is delivered outwards and the blood is pushed to the whole body. When the heart is expanding, however, will the blood in the arms and legs be drawn back to the heart like the ocean tides? If so, the blood will swarm in our blood vessels instead of remaining in its current state, and it will be impossible to achieve the interchange of materials.

If these assumptions are true and we still stand upright, the gravity will draw the blood in our veins back to the heart from positions above the heart (such as the head), which is relatively easy to be understood. However, the blood in the toes will always remain there, or wave up and down just like the tide. Since all of these do not occur in the human body, there must be a special structure to handle this issue.

This is how the human body handles this issue: the lengthwise cross section diagram of a vein in a human body is shown as follows:

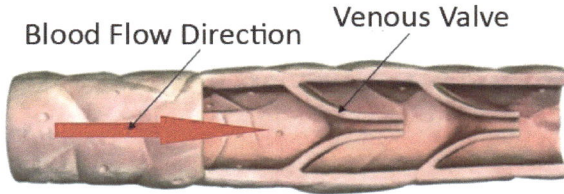

We can tell from the diagram that there is a unidirectional structure with an orientating function on the inner wall of our veins, which is called the venous valve. It can force the blood to flow along one direction by closing itself if the blood tends to flow in another direction due to gravity or other factors. Therefore the blood can be prevented from flowing from right to left in the diagram shown above.

II. BIONIC PRINCIPLE OF KINTAPE

The essential function of kintape on the human body is to change its organizational structures through controlling the flow and direction of human interstitial fluid (blood). But how can kintape control interstitial fluid? Something special will be found if we consider kintape from another perspective:

Fig. A below will be seen if we observe the kintape after its release paper is removed:

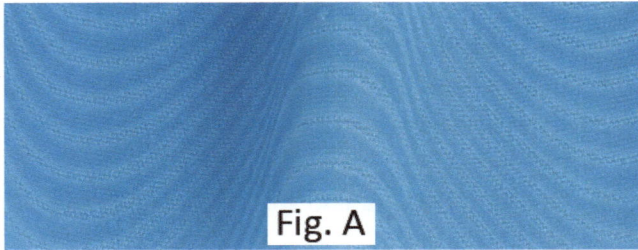

Fig. A

But when we observe from a different perspective and view the kintape from the side, we can see the structure shown in Fig. B:

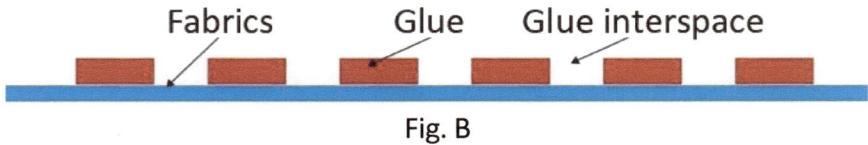

Fabrics   Glue   Glue interspace

Fig. B

When we extend the cross section along its depth (width direction of the kintape), we will find that:

1. Similar figures of Fig. B will be acquired on any longitudinal cross section; we assume and name the figures in order as Fig. B1, Fig. B2, Fig. B3, as follows:

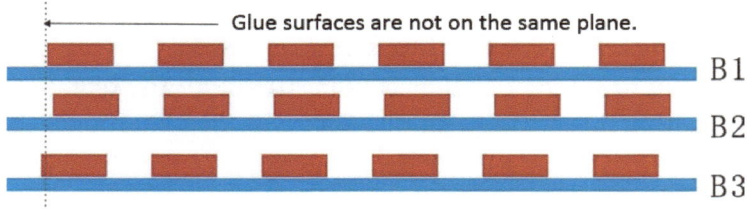

Glue surfaces are not on the same plane.

B1

B2

B3

2. On each top longitudinal section, i.e. Fig. B1, Fig. B2, two connected glue points move in one direction orderly and continuously and finally connect with each other to form a glue figure as follows:

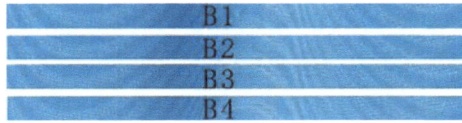

At this moment, please note that the glue bar is rectangular since no external force is changing it. Based on different production technologies and the standards of various manufacturers, the glue bar may be of other shapes. However, in spite of its form, the glue bar is vertical to fabrics, as shown in Fig. B.

Now we begin to change these glue points:

1. We stretch the kintape fully and apply it on the surface of the human body. If it is in a stationary state after applying, then Fig. C will be acquired:

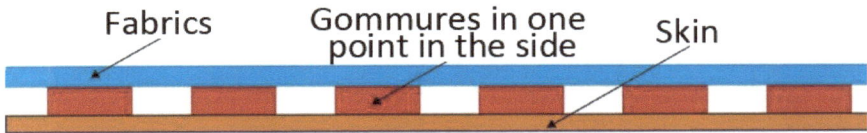

Fig. C

2. Since kintape has elastic force, it is stretched when being applied onto the skin surface. When applying onto the surface of the human body, we assume that the kintape is applied from Point A to Point B (first affix Point A, stretch the kintape toward and bond at Point B). Since kintape has rebound resilience, when the kintape is applied onto the surface of the human body and there is no external force, Fig. D below will be acquired:

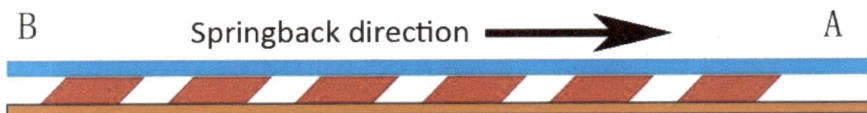

Fig. D

3. In Fig. D, the resilience force of fabrics drives the glue to deform towards one direction. Additionally, with the gluing, the skin is sufficiently firm, and the glue presses the skin, causing certain inferior fovea of the skin and driving the skin in one direction.

Fig. D1 will be acquired when enlarging the gluing point of glue and skin in Fig. D:

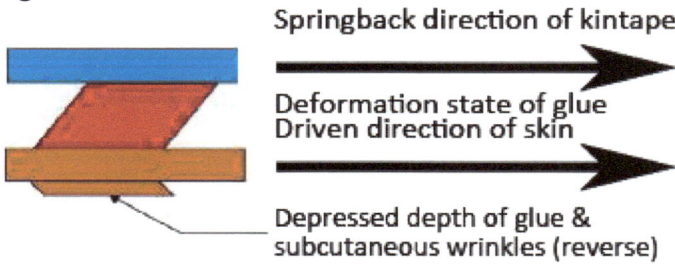

Springback direction of kintape

Deformation state of glue
Driven direction of skin

Depressed depth of glue &
subcutaneous wrinkles (reverse)

Fig. D1

4. Under the skin, the skin's form will change from Fig. D1 into Fig. E:

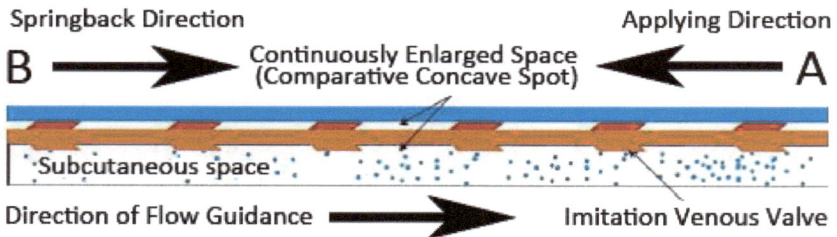

Springback Direction   Applying Direction

B ———→   Continuously Enlarged Space   ←——— A
          (Comparative Concave Spot)

Subcutaneous space

Direction of Flow Guidance ———→   Imitation Venous Valve

Fig. E

5. We can see two features in Fig. E:
   a. There are infinite structures similar to Fig. E in the width direction of the kintape. And these structures are continuous; thus the opening indicated in Fig. E will connect and form a complete channel. The channel is where middle vacant bar of glue lies;
   b. In each Fig. E, the deformed skin formed in the gluing point of the glue and skin is similar to a venous valve.

6. The subcutaneous fascia tissue of the human body is of no directivity, and the tissue fluid inside flows without order. However, as long as it flows, even if mildly, since it is beneath the skin applied with the kintape, the kintape has created:
   a. A one-way flow guidance function similar to that of a venous valve;
   b. A flowing channel of tissue fluid;

   Therefore, the tissue fluid will flow in the direction set by the kintape to change the human body. This most basic principle— and way of realizing the principle—is the origin of all functions of kintape. It accounts for basic principle of effectiveness of kintape.

III. CONSIDERATIONS OF BIOMIMETIC EFFECTIVENESS
The above section has accounted for the basic principle of kintape: bionics, which is similar to the venous valve principle of the human body. Two points shall be especially noted here:
       The first is the design and effectiveness of different forms of glue surfaces. We have mentioned many kintape products with different forms of glue surfaces in the above sections. Such products include transverse, oblique-stripe, vertical, and some so-called "air pervious" or beautiful spotted patterns. We shall understand the effectiveness of these patterns. Is it a brand-new initiative or merely a product designed blindly due to principle incomprehension, or merely designed to pursue a different appearance? Understanding this basic principle has actually indicated a promising path for product design in the future.
       Is it really effective for achieving the biomimetic principle? This point will be neglected if not considered carefully. The answer is that it is not necessarily effective even though designed according to the biomimetic principles. Therefore, in order to achieve biomimetic results, the two points below must be specified.
       Let's first assume that the product has met basic biomimetic requirements. Then what causes interaction between the kintape's imitation of a venous valve and the human body? We know that in order to make the venous valve of a human body work, there must

be pressure from the heart in blood vessels, or the venous valve is merely a one-way catheter and has no effects. Similarly, the power of kintape's effects comes from a pressure differential collected and released when the heart beats. The pressure differential causes the subcutaneous fluid pressure balance to become damaged and urges subcutaneous tissue fluid to flow. But the kintape has the features of a venous valve and can activate the subcutaneous tissue fluid creating a flow in a set direction. To keep its smooth flow, kintape requires certain technical standards and specific parameter requirements, so as to achieve maximum integration with the functions of the human body. This requires further optimization of the technical parameters of kintape.

To achieve the maximum effect and address the above questions, we will discuss the two points below from a perspective of technology.

The first is fabric. It should be as thick and elastic as that of the skin it is to be applied on, so as to achieve optimum compatibility with the skin. But how thick and elastic is the skin? The skin of a human body varies. Even for the same person, the thickness and elastic force of skin varies in different locations, and cannot be predicted, so a standard had to be created for our products that would most closely fit needed specifications. Therefore, in 2011, to ensure the prevention of fabrics from meshing (too sparse or too dense), I set basic specifications for gray fabric all-cotton kintape as: (21s + 70D) × 16s/34 × 38. Let me explain the meaning of the row of figures: (21s + 70D) indicates that the kintape warp yarns are 21 cotton yarns with a 70D spandex filament wrapped in the core (core spun). [It shall be particularly noted that the larger the number of cotton yarn is, the thinner the yarn is. The larger D (Denier) is, the thicker the spandex filament is. These figures will be referred to in the following context with the same meaning]. Weft yarns are 16 cotton yarns, and 34 × 38 indicates that within one inch (one inch for warp and weft yarns) there are 34 warp yarns and 38 weft ones, all calculated based on a fully-stretched specification. Meanwhile, the standard of elastic force is specified as 1:1.6. Luckily, this is also the current global standard. However, the standard has one problem: it has ensured that the product cannot be thinly dispersed to meet it.

Meanwhile, the gram weight of gray fabric is nearly 200 g/m^2, which is obviously thicker and harder. When used on certain locations (e.g. wrist and waist), it will cause incomplete bonding or the position may feel pricking after it having been applied for a while. To test, I applied the product where the skin surface area is largest, bent it to its minimum area after applying, and saw the bonding of fabrics and skin from one side and experienced the somatic sense. Therefore, in 2012, I specified the gram weight of finished fabrics as 165±5 g/m^2 to make it softer and more fitting by reducing the quantity of fabric and nearly 35 g/m^2 on the surface (refer to patent for invention: Warp and Weft Shredded Sport Kintape and its Manufacturing Method, ZL 2012 1 0133773.8). Hence, the fabrics are closer to the skin's thickness, and the softness is also closer to that of skin. Now warp and weft shredding has become a standard parameter for all manufacturers.

Essentially speaking, it is certain that the performance and somatic sense will be better when the fabrics become thinner and are closer to the skin's characteristics. When writing this book and considering other factors (e.g. production technology, operational convenience of product and current production technology conditions), I have tried my best to determine an industrialization level. Products closer to skin are still under trial-manufacturing, but I believe more professional manufacturers will produce better products with manufacturer improvements and the efforts made by various manufacturers.

The second point is about glue. Development of glue can be divided into the following parts:

1. TYPES OF GLUE:

Before 2010, medical hot melt glue was mainly used for kintape products. In 2010, I established several small rehabilitation centers for trial use. I found that the effects of using medical hot melt glue were not satisfactory. First, it is about treatment effects; second, it is about the bonding duration. Generally, the glue may not keep its bonding for more than 24 hours and has poor waterproofing. Practical cases may require a bonding duration of more than 7 days

(168 hours). In that very year, we required that only medical acrylic acid shall be used. The viscosity and waterproofing as well as the effects of medical acrylic acid are completely superior to those of hot melt glue. Nowadays, medical acrylic acid is the most common glue used all over the world in kintape products.

2. VISCOSITY:

The national viscosity standard of common tapes is 0.9 N/CM, a standard obviously unavailable except for paper tapes for intravenous drip or normal sport tapes. In 2012, we specified the viscosity standard as 2.5 N/CM, which has become the basic standard of kintape products globally. But actually, the standard retains bonding for nearly 48 hours only, which is still reasonable given the actual technological production level of other manufacturers. However, with increased research on kintape in the past two years as well as the innovation of glue and manufacturing techniques, in 2015 we improved our production standard to 5 N/CM to increase the length of bonding (it is only limited to self-owned brands and several limited global cooperative brands).

3. GRAM WEIGHT OF GLUE (DRY GLUE WEIGHT):

So far there is no uniform global standard. But the value shall be related to two parameters, i.e. the larger the gram weight of the glue in each square meter is, the better the viscosity will be. The second is about the closeness to the subcutaneous fascia tissue fluid in the human body. Since we are unable to understand or research the molecular weight of fascia tissue fluid in the human body, in order to improve the closeness and viscosity effects, we specified 65 ± 5 g/m^2 in 2013. The value is certainly not the optimum. Based on my trial use in over ten thousand cases, however, effects are still much higher than 50 g/m^2 specified previously or 35 g/m^2 for some manufacturers. The value still requires further research by more professional experts to perfect product functions and to improve efficiency.

From the above sections, we can make a summary and further specify kintape elements. For example, the fundamental principle of the function implementation of kintape is the imitation of the venous valve principle of the human body. We can also make circulating tissue fluid smoother and larger, provided that the features of the fabrics and glue are close to those of the skin and the subcutaneous fascia tissue fluid in the human body respectively. The glue shall meet actual requirement for usage which is mainly reflected in the viscosity standard.

PART II:
SIX FUNCTIONAL PRINCIPLES

In Part I, we explained the fundamental principle of kintape: bionics. The degree of understanding of this basic principle directly influences:

1. The product process technology and design principle; for functional requirements, it rejects fabrics or arabesquitic glue products that lack the imitation of the venous valve effects.
2. The directive guidance for application position and operation techniques during usage only explains the proposition of why kintape serves the human body. It has no operability yet and is insufficient to understand the strong functions of kintape. It cannot serve as a guiding principle in direct use of kintape.
3. Basic product standard, including requirements for fabrics and glue. In this way, for practicality, kintape also has six functional principles. Users may not judge use independently and should adjust usage during operation unless they have a good command of the six principles.

1. FLOW GUIDANCE

Flow guidance is the top function among all six functional principles as it is directly derived from the basic principle of imitation of the venous valve effects and will be used in treating muscles, nerves, blood, lymph, etc. It can be said that it is one of the most widely-used principles. Sometimes, even if it seems that other functional principles have played its role, the proper results cannot be implemented without the basic function of flow guidance. The reasons and methods of producing flow guidance are to bond a kintape similar to the human skin on the human body's surface, making the glue surface produce one-way effects similar to a venous valve through certain techniques, then change subcutaneous wrinkles through the one-way wrinkle, and make the static tissue fluid of the human body flow through the pressure difference produced by the heart, specifying the moving direction of current tissue fluid according to the direction set by the imitation of the venous valve.

Here we will outline the effects of flow guidance:

Fascia tissue lies beneath the skin of a human body. It is similar in form to sponge and full of tissue fluid containing blood, neurons, and lymph, as well as inflammations that may cause discomfort. In a normal state, the tissue fluid in fascia tissue is not circulating or is circulating disorderly. This so-called disordered circulation indicates the circulation of the tissue fluid has no directivity. When inflammations exist in tissue fluid and the circulation of tissue fluid has no directivity, lymph, the self-defense tissue of the human body, may not reach the site where inflammations exist. Therefore, if we can provide a circulation direction and force for the tissue fluid, we can accelerate or improve the transmission of lymph to the inflammation site and remove inflammation faster. In certain positions, if the lymph is completely static or unreachable, the inflammation may be removed even though it is difficult to do so.

We often see some old people who have suffered lymph gland necrosis for various reasons, causing various injuries and inflammation of the surrounding tissue. We can utilize the flow guidance to connect the inflammation site with other complete lymph glands and form an effective introduction to the lymph gland.

The way of achieving the flow guidance is generally to affix and apply one end of the kintape, then stretch it to the other end gently and apply evenly.

Three aspects shall be noted particularly:
1. When bonding in the other direction from B to the affixed end A, the circulation direction of tissue fluid is from B to A.
2. Under all circumstances, it must be ensured that the tissue fluid circulates from lymph glands to the inflammation site. Reverse circulation is not allowed. This is mainly because we often cannot tell whether bacterial inflammation or non-bacterial ones are causing the discomfort. Opposite operation may cause the enlargement of the lymph gland as the inflammation damages lymph glands.

3. Do not affix one end first and then stretch the kintape fully before applying it onto the body surface, as this may fail to achieve flow guidance. Please stretch the kintape during the process of applying. Users can build a model for analysis according to the below schematic diagram.

The functional schematic diagram is as follows:

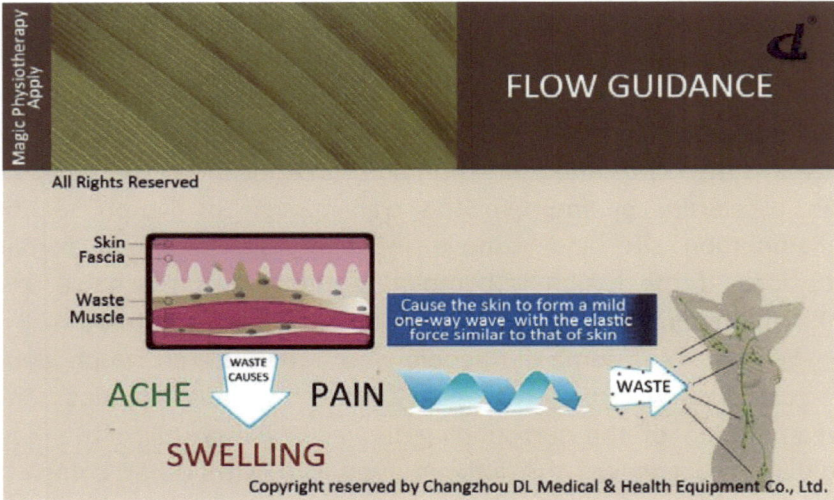

Magic Physiotherapy Apply

FLOW GUIDANCE

Skin
Fascia

Waste
Muscle

Cause the skin to form a mild one-way wave with the elastic force similar to that of skin

ACHE   WASTE CAUSES   PAIN   WASTE

SWELLING

2. PROMOTING BLOOD CIRCULATION

The kintape has effective flow guidance effects on the tissue fluid if used correctly. If we decide to use it mainly for blood, we can change to a certain degree the blood flow direction as shown in Fig. A:

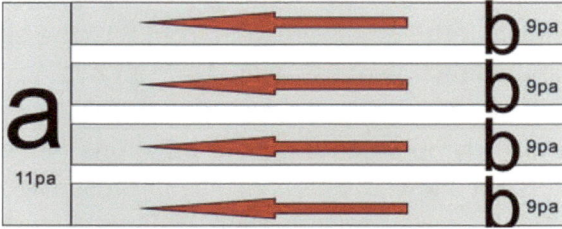

a

11pa

b 9pa
b 9pa
b 9pa
b 9pa

Fig. A

In Fig. A, we can see that the blood forms a flow guidance along Point b to Point a. Assume that the blood pressure of the position to be applied is 10 pa and relatively static before applying the kintape. After applying the kintape—as the flow guidance is thereby formed—we can easily understand that Point a and Point b in Fig. A must have a difference in blood pressure. The blood pressure of Point a shall be higher than that of Point b (e.g. 11 pa in Point a while 9 pa in Point b). In this example, since the blood pressure of Point b is lower than that of Point a, there are two possibilities. First, the blood of Point a returns to Point b. However, based on the first principle (principle of venous valve), the blood cannot acquire the same amount of backflow. If this is impossible, Point b must absorb and supplement blood from positions other than the applied site to keep the blood pressure balance. But for Point a, as the blood pressure of the applied site is higher than that of sites with no kintape applied, Point a will have an overflow effect and blood circulation will be created. At this time, theoretically speaking, the blood may flow as shown in Fig. A1:

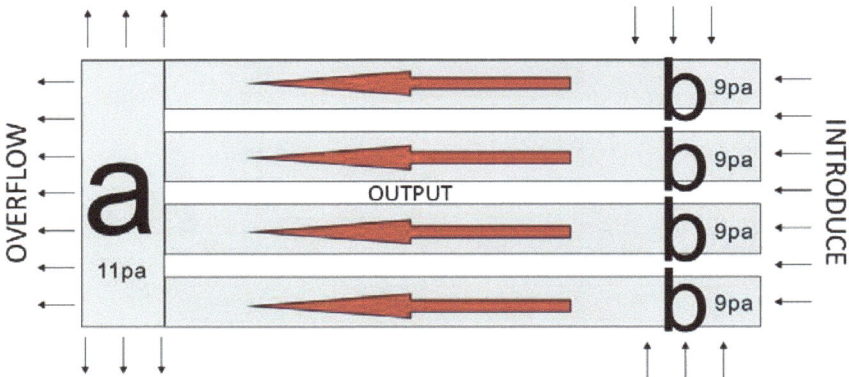

Fig. A1

Arrows in Fig. A, A1, and B indicate the flow direction of blood. If we are simply describing the realization of blood circulation in Fig. A and Fig. A1, then in Fig. B we can see a very complex schematic diagram of blood circulation. It shall be noted that Fig. B only describes a flow diagram of blood at one point in time. In fact, due to the complexity of the human body, even the heartbeat will cause pressure values to change ceaselessly and blood circulation paths will be more complex and precise. However, subcutaneous blood circulation in a certain point has been realized and the circulation will promote blood changes in deeper levels of muscles.

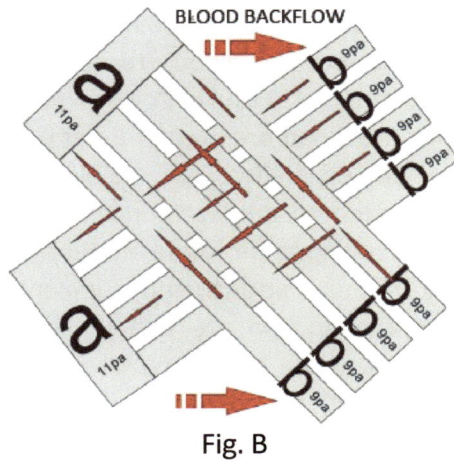

Fig. B

Acceleration of blood circulation can promote the improvement of blood oxygen content for one position: remove extravasated blood, realize detumescence (reduction of swelling), recover ossified/rigid muscles, etc. The original diagram is as follows:

3. SORTING OUT FASCIA TISSUE

Previously, we had mentioned fascia tissue while discussing flow guidance. There is a large amount of liquid in fascia, which is collectively referred to as tissue fluid with fluidity. The fascia tissue is in a network shape and has no orientation in itself. When the body is in a normal state, the non-orientation of fascia tissue may not be a problem, but if the circulation of tissue fluid is blocked or a large amount of inflammation exists in the tissue fluid, the waste generated by metabolism will not be discharged from the body timely and effectively. This causes our bodies to become sore. If the tissue fluid in fascia tissue can flow based on our needs and spontaneously form a circulating habit, it will then effectively improve our human body system and spontaneously eliminate inflammation. Therefore, it is one of the functional principles of kintape.

The method of sorting out fascia tissue is similar to that of blood circulation, however the purposes are different. In blood circulation, the main purpose is to achieve blood circulation under the body surface, and to thereby lead the blood circulation in a deeper level. While in sorting out fascia tissue, the purpose is to establish a channel for the circulation of tissue fluid and to make it form a habitual channel. The target objects are the orientation and route of circulation of tissue fluid. In many cases of practical operation, it is to the user's benefit to use the same method as that of blood circulation and achieve both functions.

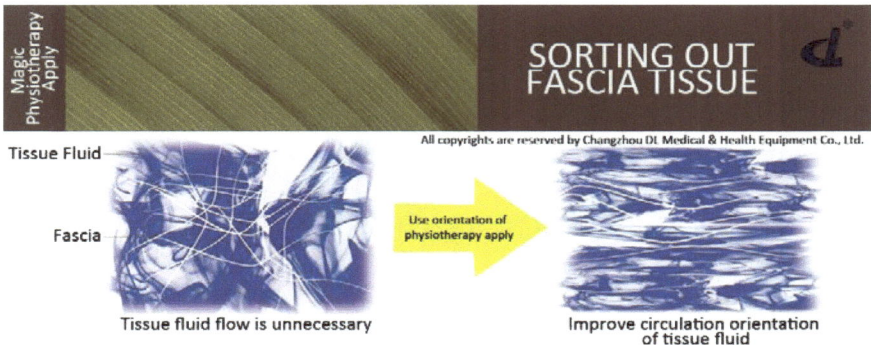

Magic Physiotherapy Apply

SORTING OUT FASCIA TISSUE

Tissue Fluid

Fascia

Use orientation of physiotherapy apply

Tissue fluid flow is unnecessary

Improve circulation orientation of tissue fluid

4. ACUPUNCTURE POINTS EFFECT

In the traditional Chinese medical (TCM) system, there are many acupoints in the human body, and each has a different significance. The purpose of this book, however, is not to remember or understand the functions of all of the different acupoints, but is instead to make sure that everybody can master and skillfully use kintape. Therefore, we can understand acupoints in human bodies in the following respects.

If the human body is a complex traffic route map, then these acupoints are key points on each expressway or city street. They have their respective routes, with mutual non-interference, but interact with each other. If a certain point in this general map goes wrong (e.g. becoming blocked), in the theory of TCM, it can be adjusted through acupoints, analogous to a restaurant, gas station, or toll station along the way. In other words, when we take a look at the Diagram of Human Acupoints (located at the front of the book), all acupoints can be deemed as energy or material exchange points on different parts (or routes) in the human bodies. When we adjust these energy exchange points, it is the equivalent to adjusting the corresponding part or circulation route of the body, and thus realizing the purpose of adjustment of the human body.

But it is indeed very difficult to remember such a large amount of acupoints and to understand the logical relations among them. Maybe it cannot be achieved until the end of our lives. So we utilize the powerful function of kintape, and manufacture or create energy exchanges ourselves.

As we discussed the theories on flow guidance and blood circulation, we understand that kintape has those two functions. Now, if we apply kintape on the human body as per Fig. C, we will find out that the blood or tissue fluid at Point a will flow toward Point b, while the blood or tissue fluid at Point c will also flow toward Point b. Then, we can assume that the thing flowing from a to b is tissue fluid with a large quantity of lymph fluid starting from lymphoglandula, while the thing flowing from c to b is the inflammatory factor causing the human body to be sore. They converge at Point b, and Point b forms an exchange point of lymph fluid and inflammation. This creates the function that we require from acupoints, i.e. the function of exchanging energy or material. It is also equivalent to creating a new acupoint with the function of exchanging energy or material on the surface of the human body. This is the acupuncture point's effect.

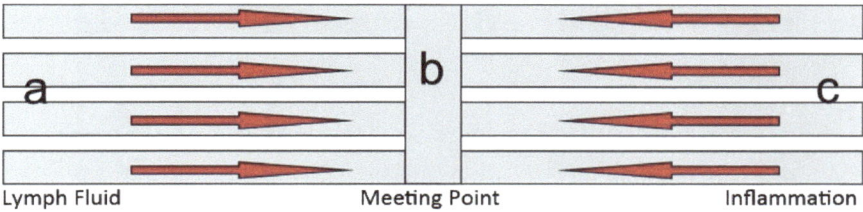

Fig. C

In practical use, it is unnecessary to achieve symmetry in energy exchange or while using the taping method. Even in applying from one end to another, the pressure differential will generate from one end and thus force the material exchange of tissue fluid under the applied part. This is similar to flow guidance, blood circulation, or the smoothing of fascia tissue. In the same way, however, the four things stress on different points. In the principle of acupoints, it focuses on the forced material exchange of the damaged point and thus accelerates the recovery of the damaged point.

Likewise, when blood or tissue fluid flows to a certain point by force, the blood vessel or nerve being closed or blocked can be opened up. And we can understand this point as one of the acupoints in the human body.

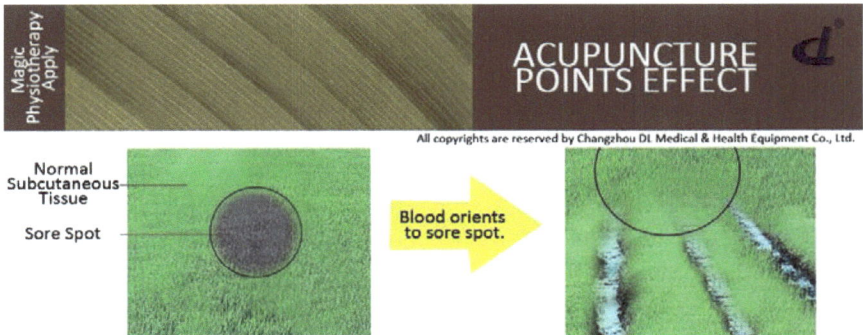

5. INTENSIFY OR RELAX MUSCLE TISSUE

This theory is widely used and accepted in the practical use of kintape. It is mainly because this point is the easiest to be understood, and can also be easily mastered in practice. For this point, we will not discuss how many human muscles there are or the operation modes of each muscle or muscle group. What we focus on is to explain the convenience of operation.

Below the skin, there is subcutaneous muscle tissue. Muscle has a certain directivity and because of this, the human body can achieve relaxation or intensification and thus perform different actions such as bowing and stretching, grabbing and dropping, and bending and straightening.

The human body as we understand it is a mechanical structure with supporting points. No matter what actions we perform, there is a supporting point and lift. In the case where the supporting point does not move, no matter whether we lift or lower, certain muscles or muscle groups must perform the process of shrinking or stretching. This process of shrinking or stretching is the process of intensification and relaxation of the muscle. When intensifying (lifting), if we intend to bear more strength, we must provide great strength support to the shrinking (bearing strength) muscle group. Since the kintape has shrinking force, if the direction of shrinking is the same as that of the shrinking of muscle, then it will generate intensification of the muscle, otherwise muscle relaxation can be achieved.

In practical use, if we have understood the principle mentioned above, we will find that in the process of achieving muscle intensification, the theory of blood circulation is also achieved in the same taping method, even though muscle intensification comes from a different principle.

When the muscle constantly repeats movements in a certain way or is damaged by external mechanical forces, or when the endured strength exceeds the endurance limit of muscle, the muscle will be in a tense or "loss of strength" state, presenting soreness, spasms, and stiffness. By applying the kintape along or against the trend of the muscle, muscle intensification or relaxation can be achieved.

In the use of this theory, there are two difficult problems. First, distinguishing the muscle group. Sometimes, intensification of one part of a muscle group will cause the relaxation of its adjacent muscle group if the user is are not being able to distinguish the edge of the muscle group and thus applies the kintape too far, and vice versa. Therefore, the edge of each muscle group must be remembered. Of course, the simplest way is to have a Diagram of Human Muscles (located at the front of the book) close at hand. Second, judging the direction of human muscles can be difficult. When it is impossible to distinguish if a certain muscle is intensifying or relaxing, a mnemonic method is not completely right, however it can represent the directions of most muscles of the human body as given here:

1. Stand normally.
2. Take all joints as the starting points; applying kintape from the joints downwards is for intensification (however, do not apply on the lower half of muscle group), and applying from the joints upwards is for relaxation.
3. Take the body's vertical middle line (vertebration) as the starting point; applying toward the two sides is for intensification, and applying from the two sides toward the center is for relaxation.
4. Take the painful vertebra as the starting point; applying downward is for intensification, and upward for relaxation.

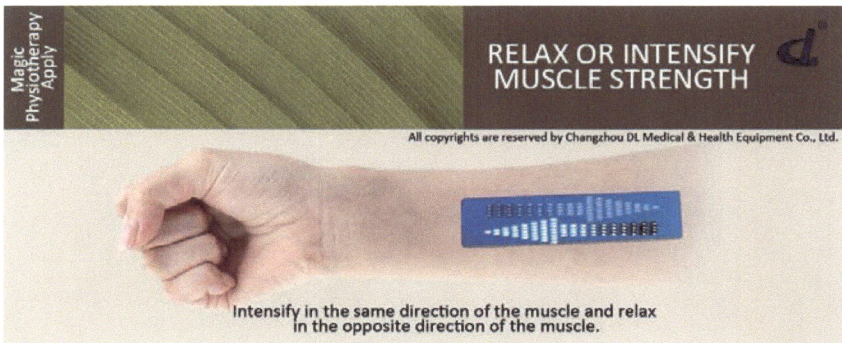

Magic Physiotherapy Apply

RELAX OR INTENSIFY MUSCLE STRENGTH

Intensify in the same direction of the muscle and relax in the opposite direction of the muscle.

6. GATE CONTROL THEORY

Gate control theory is used to explain the reason that pain reduces with the use of kintape. For example, when a child cries after getting an injection on the arm, the parent usually carries him/her in the bosom and caresses him/her on the back and bottom. However, they often don't caresses the place that was pricked by the needle, yet the child will stop crying gradually. Why? Does the child stop feeling the pain?

In fact, that is not the case. The child stops crying because the number of nerves with pain existing in the fascia is much less than the number of nerves that carry the sense of the touching to the skin by foreign objects, and the speed of the transferring signal by the touched nerve is much higher than that of the pained nerve. In unit area, when giving a greater number and concentration of stimulation to the touched nerve, if the number of nerve signals flowing toward the brain is consistent, the number of pain nerves flowing towards the brain will be diluted. And thus the pain will reduce or disappear.

The applying and covering functions of the kintape is just like increasing the stimulation from foreign objects touching the skin. Closing the transferring number of pain nerves, the high elasticity of the kintape will further enhance the feeling capacity of the skin and so further enhance the proportion of the transferred touch sensation to the brain. It has a strong practical significance in a wide range of pain with unknown causes.

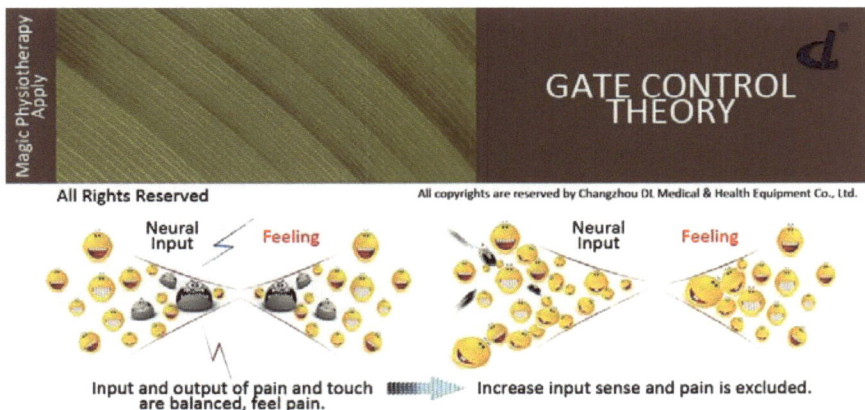

Magic Physiotherapy Apply

GATE CONTROL THEORY

Neural Input | Feeling

Neural Input | Feeling

Input and output of pain and touch are balanced, feel pain. Increase input sense and pain is excluded.

After understanding the above mentioned six principles, there is a critical problem—although not specifically a principle—that must be further understood.

We have previously mentioned that the primary applied principle of kintape is flow guidance. Although in the respect of basic principles, it is based on bionics, there is an important element of flow guidance: the establishment of the channel. If there is no subcutaneous channel, flow guidance cannot be achieved. So there is an important function of kintape: the enhancement of subcutaneous space by applying the kintape on the surface of the skin through certain techniques, creating stretching or shrinking on certain parts of the skin so as to enhance the stretching part and to enlarge the subcutaneous space.

You can practice through the following method: cut off an X-shaped piece (with the length of about 10 cm) and find an entirely flat piece of paper. Under a fully loose status, apply the X in the middle of the paper, and then pull the 4 corners of the X diagonally. Soon you will find that the middle point of the X is enhanced and the paper is sagged. This example is typical. In practical use, when combined with the appropriate techniques, any shape of kintape can achieve this function. The reason we don't incorporate this into the principles is that different operating methods will cause different results. It will be broken down in the subsequent technique part.

PART III:
ACTION PRINCIPLES & INTERRELATION OF PRODUCT PARAMETERS

So far, we have discussed the six basic principles as to why kintape can achieve its functions as well as the theoretical explanation for the interrelation that can be formed between kintape and the human body in order to improve the human body's functions. Since products shall be used to achieve those functions, we are going to further explain the previous functional parameters of products and their specific changes in detail:

I. ELASTIC FORCE

The elastic force referred to here has two meanings: First, it refers to the largest length of skin increased from natural length in cases of transformation resulting from longitudinal stress. For convenience, it is hereinafter referred to as the elastic force rate. Second, it refers to the strength required to pull open the kintape longitudinally, which stands for the strength that may be generated during the retraction of kintape, which is hereinafter referred to as the elastic force value to distinguish these two meanings.

THE FUNCTIONS AND OBJECTIVES OF THE ELASTIC FORCE RATE:

We've already mentioned issues concerning specifying standard values for elastic force. I'd like to talk about the derivation of the elastic force of kintape first.

In the initial phase of kintape application (before 2010 or so), the elastic force value of products was generally 1:1.2 or 1:1.4. The reason is that at the time, the objective of using kintape was to bind up joints or muscles. A certain pressing force is very important for the kintape, as poor affixation effects will be generated if the elastic force rate is too high. Therefore products at that time tended to be a median between heavy and light bandages. During the application of kintape, however, people began to realize that it might impose a greater influence on muscles, even greater than that on joint protection. The elastic force value (1:1.2 or 1:1.4) could not meet relevant requirements if it was applied to muscles.

In 2010, we took the first step to select five manufacturing standards, namely 1:1.2, 1:1.4, 1:1.6, 1:1.8 and 1:2.0. We also applied them in our own recovery stores for comparison. Practical application indicated that when the elastic force rate was lower than 1:1.4, the operator might feel an obvious lack of elastic force. When the elastic force rate was 1:1.8 or higher, however, insufficient supporting force would be provided for certain applications. 1:1.6 was determined to be a compatible rate for both elastic force and supporting force. After several years of development, the main elastic force standard for kintape is defined as 1:1.6. What are the advantages of this rate? First, it is compatible with the requirements of higher rates, such as that of over 1:1.8 for skin on the crooks of joints, providing proper supporting force and affixation. Second, it is compatible with the requirements of lower rates, such as that of about 1:1.4 for skin on the body surface, and can provide a certain supporting force.

To emphasize the application requirements and prevent improper application as much as possible, since negative effects are mainly caused by many people not being aware of the strong effects of kintape, which will be discussed later in this section, we have defined the application scope standard for the elastic force of the kintape. When it is applied to medical treatment, the tensile strength is 1:1.2; sports, 1:1.4; first aid, 1:1.6.

The reason for these application scopes are as follows:
1. The fundamental objective of elastic force is to induce the imitation venous valve effect in skin through retraction. The tensile strength will directly influence the venous valve effects and when cooperating with other manufacturing parameters, the strength of flow guidance or other functions. However, since the bearable range of the human body is limited, restrictions must be imposed on it.
2. Elastic force rate and value directly influence the sensations of the human body. When they are combined with the six fundamental principles, we may find that the elastic force rate is always an important factor that influences every change in the human body.

3. Different application scopes and parts exist in recovery, including common diseases, the treatment of sports injuries and protection, muscle strength, and first aid. Therefore, the application time and influences on the skin are also different. Skin tends to be pulled till injured if the same program is selected for all instances.
4. Essentially, a product can be similar to skin only if it is equipped with elastic force. Products without elastic force are not able to deliver functions in accordance with those of skin.

Based on changes of values in elastic force, we may conclude that the elastic force rate of 1:1.4 is sufficient only for sports products (such as those for increasing or releasing the strength of muscles, fastening joints and limiting curvature), and 1:1.6 is suitable for circumstances requiring more functions. Of course, when 1:1.6 is selected, more requirements will exist for the proficiency of operators, too.

IMPLEMENTATION METHODS OF ELASTIC FORCE CONTROL:
In practical application, the operators cannot control the tensile strength accurately themselves, and they will usually believe the tensile strength they have imposed is insufficient. Practical tests show that taking commonly skilled users as the criteria, the accuracy is about 20% accuracy in ten tests for tensile strength control. This is a striking percentage. That's why many symptoms similar to irritability will occur, often appearing first on skin. One also may sometimes feel itching with subcutaneous extravasated blood points. In practical operation, over 90% users will suffer from over-stretching after the kintape is applied for a certain time (usually about 24 hours). We provide two operation programs to this end:

1. Requirements for the release degree of the release paper: i.e. the adhesive force between the release paper and fabric. The control standard is that the stretching rate of kintape is about 20% in the case that the fabric is not stretched and the kintape is stretched naturally after one of its ends is applied onto the skin. A stretching rate of about 20% can be obtained when kintape is applied to the

therapeutic process. It shall be noted that this is only the standard for Changzhou DL Medical & Health Equipment Co., Ltd. rather than other manufacturers, thus it is not suitable to assume this standard for the products of other manufacturers. We'd like to invite all manufacturers to set this as the universal manufacturing standard to provide convenience for users.

2. To print or weave patterns (one of them is a little soccer ball-shaped pattern) on the surfaces of products (refer to the patent for the invention of Changzhou DL Medical & Health Equipment Co., Ltd.: ZL 2012 2 0279940.5). The application method: When the little soccer ball is pulled to a perfect circle, the tensile strength is about 120%; when the hexagon in the middle is pulled to a regular shape, 140%; when the little soccer ball is pulled completely, 160%. As shown in the Fig. below:

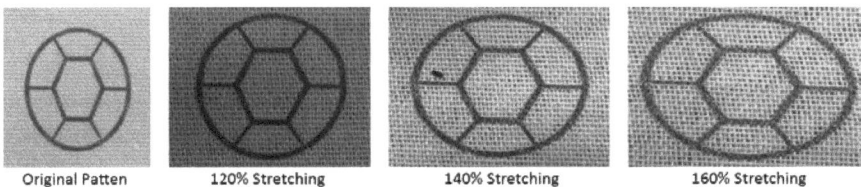

| Original Patten | 120% Stretching | 140% Stretching | 160% Stretching |

II. WIDTH OF GLUE SURFACE

With the understanding of the previous principle of the basic origin of kintape, we may easily understand that the width of glue surface is a parameter of great importance, rather than insignificant or for manufacturing only.

After the kintape is applied onto the surface of the human body, it is the glue to which the human body is exposed. A downward pressure will be formed after the glue is applied onto the surface of the human body and conducted into the subcutaneous area. It will make the skin recess downward, cooperating with the elastic force (springback) to form subcutaneous structures similar to that of venous valves. Thus the width of the glue surface in fact determines that of the subcutaneous structure. From this perspective, the wider the glue surface is, the wider the imitation venous valve is and the faster the flow guidance is. With the same width of the glue surface, the larger the tensile strength of the fabric is, the faster the flow guidance is due to the shortened circulation distance.

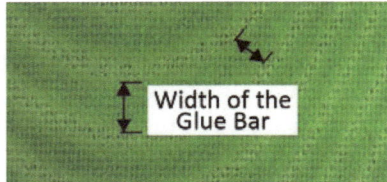

Width of the
Glue Bar

III. WIDTH OF OPENINGS ON KINTAPE GLUE BARS

The opening on a kintape glue bars refers to the middle part of wave-shaped glue surfaces without glue. We have learned from previous sections that the opening in the middle part of glue bar is equal to the middle opening between two venous valves in the imitation venous valve structures. When the kintape is applied onto the human body, the opening will bulge compared to the glue surface. The more it bulges, the wider it and the subcutaneous space will be. Thus, it cannot be designed to be too wide so as to prevent the flow guidance from being too fast for the human body to bear, especially when the flow is guided from the bottom to the top. Additionally, it cannot be designed to be too narrow, either. It should be thicker than the sunken area resulting from the pressure imposed on skin by the glue bar, or it will be impossible to conduct flow guidance.

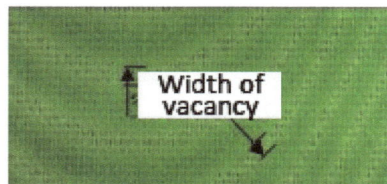

Width of
vacancy

IV. SIZE OF RIPPLE CYCLE

The size of ripple cycle refers to the length of fabric covered by one cycle of the waves on the glue surface. It involves the distance of blood flow in the same length. The shorter the distance is, the larger the flow of interstitial fluid (per unit time) and the stronger the sensation of the human body will be. Likewise, if the flow is too large and exceeds the bearable range for skin, or for the human body, it will cause harm. If the flow is too small, the functions will not be obvious.

To this end, more attention shall be paid in the product design. We are far off a perfect parameter, and efforts will be made continuously in order to pursue a favorable program for most people.

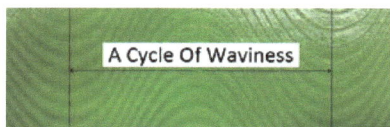

A Cycle Of Waviness

V. THICKNESS OF FABRIC

We have mentioned before that every effort should be made to ensure the fabric is closer to skin. This is not only an issue with the compatibility of fabric with skin, but also an important program to achieve the smooth flow guidance. In addition, the closer to skin the fabric is, the greater the fit will be achieved when applying. Great fit is a basic requirement to achieve the six principles mentioned before. Flow guidance and acupuncture points effect will be impossible if the kintape cannot fit the skin. If the fit is not correct, the only functions it may then deliver will be increasing or releasing the strength of muscles.

VI. FUNCTIONS OF VISCOSITY

We have mentioned that the stronger the viscosity, the greater the fit between the kintape and the human body, and the longer the applied time will be (the larger the strength against springback will be). Glue has another important function in addition to the physical functions above, which is the reason the requirements for the gram weight of glue are enhanced. After being applied onto the human body, every glue bar will press the skin downward to form a recessed area on the skin through which the structure of the venous valve can be created. The length of a venous valve is closely relevant to the thickness (perpendicular to the fabric) of the glue bar. The thicker the glue bar is, the greater the pressure imposed and the longer the venous valve will be, achieving greater effects. Therefore, theoretically the gram weight of glue can be further increased. Limited by the relation between the holes of fabric and the viscosity of glue, however, we can at present only set 70 g/m^2 as an approximate safe value to prevent the glue from permeating to the rear of the product. Of course, since technical progress has an unlimited future, it is believed that after understanding the basic theory, more enterprises will manage to develop better technologies to continuously improve the quality and applicability of products.

VII. OPERATION METHOD

It is not difficult for us to understand the importance of the operation method based on the product's technical aspects discussed previously, which can be summarized as follows:

1. The tensile value of elastic force for medical treatment is 120%; for sports, 140%; and for first aid, 160%. For an acute sprain, for example, the tensile value of 120% can be achieved by pulling the paper. And others may be achieved through the experience or indicative marks on the product surface.
2. For products of the same type, the larger the tensile strength is, the faster the flow guidance will be.
3. For glue of the same gram weight, the greater the viscosity, the stronger the ability of the glue to change the skin and the lower the requirements for tensile strength.
4. The thinner the fabric, the lower the tensile strength needed as kintape tends to be over-pulled unintentionally.
5. The smaller the ripple cycle, the shorter the distance of simultaneous interstitial fluid flow. The greater tensile range is required to achieve more obvious effects, but what the human body can bear must be considered.
6. The healthier the person (i.e. the stronger the ability of blood circulation is), the stronger his ability to bear tensile strength. On the contrary, the stronger the tensile strength, the more obvious the sensation.

Operation methods relevant to applicability will be discussed in detail in the methods to achieve each function later.

CHAPTER III: TAPING METHODS

PART I:
BASIC KNOWLEDGE FOR STRUCTURES OF HUMAN BODY

Kintape mainly acts on the blood, lymph, nerves, muscles, and meridians of the human body. Here, I'd like to provide a brief introduction to their overall principles, based on the structure diagram of the systems of the human body (please refer to the figures attached at the beginning on the book):

I. BLOOD

The overall direction of blood flow: from the heart to each part of the human body (through the arteries) and then back to the heart (through the veins). Thus, to accelerate the return of blood to the heart, the starting point of kintape shall be applied near the heart and the terminal away from the heart. This will make the returning blood flow along the direction of the blood in the veins so that the blood's circulation can be accelerated and the oxygen content of the blood can be increased.

II. LYMPH

Lymph is an important protection system of the human body. When treating non-bacterial inflammation and removing acid materials through kintape, the lymphatic system will generally be used. The lymphatic system, however, is a little different from the blood circulation system. To understand the lymph, we may compare it to an army: the heart is the general lymph node, which is equal to the supreme headquarters of an army. This supreme headquarters will send soldiers to each joint of the human body, which are lymph nodes. Additionally, every region in the area within jurisdiction of the whole army requires a reconnaissance team, which is the lymphatic system distributed throughout the whole body. The transportation system that conducts army transfer is the lymphatic fluid.

Since this is a progressive system, in most cases in handling problems relevant to inflammation, the lymphatic fluid will be exported from positions adjacent to lymph nodes and imported to the inflammatory parts. It is aimed at increasing the density of lymph fluid and eliminating inflammation. As previously mentioned, in cases of handling problems relevant to inflammation, the main method is to introduce lymph fluid rather than introducing the inflammation to the lymph, since the type of inflammation (bacterial or non-bacterial) cannot be determined. Theoretically, better anti-inflammatory results would be achieved if we import the inflammation to lymph nodes, but that would pose potential risks and safety shall be given priority. We do not know whether lymph inflammation would be caused with the entrance of bacterial inflammation (e.g. viral inflammation) to lymph nodes.

Another common problem that may arise when we handle problems related to the lymph is that many patients may suffer from lymph node necrosis (e.g. lymph node necrosis may occur in the knee in cases of rheumatoid arthritis). Lymphatic fluid import from the ankle or inguinal lymph nodes may be considered in this regard.

III. MUSCLE AND LIGAMENT

In Chapter II, we discussed the directivity of muscles. In fact, it is very difficult to subdivide the directivity of each muscle. Each action of the human body is collaboratively completed by many muscle groups, including intensive and relaxed muscle groups. If we can handle each muscle based on the specific condition of each different individual, a satisfactory effect will then be achieved. In practical use, however, the muscle group of each consumer is not standard. In operational details, moreover, each muscle group cannot achieve the capacity of independent handling. Therefore, we just need to memorize the alignment graphics in the general muscles drawing, which can make memorizing easy. In summary, taking each joint as a demarcation point, apply from the top down to intensify strength, apply from the bottom up to relax strength; taking the spine as the trunk line, apply from the middle outward to intensify strength, apply from the outside inward to relax strength; taking the back spine as an intermediate point, apply from the top down to intensify strength, and apply from the bottom up to relax strength.

In practical use, muscles are often used. Some of the frequently-used principles and the following problems are noted here:

1. Pay attention to the dialectical relationship of intensifying and relaxing strength. For example: for aching shoulders, would it be more beneficial to intensify or relax strength? It depends. Many operators discover that both intensifying and relaxing strength are effective to consumers who will however claim that there are no effects after a while, or it is intensified. Why? That is because different discomforts may be caused by different situations. Taking aches in the shoulders as an example: if it is caused by moving heavy objects, it can be judged as insufficient strength and strength needs to be intensified. But if the muscle has been torn, relaxing strength would be needed, as well as wrapping properly. If it is an accumulation injury of caused by strain (e.g. incorrect sitting posture), strength needs to be relaxed. If tearing pain has formed, intensify strength for the first time, while relaxing strength for the second time if needed. Of course, we still need to take other factors into consideration to make a judgment.
2. Muscle issues caused by special cases cannot be handled simply according to intensification or relaxation, which mainly include the following situations:
   a. Intensification shall be adopted for muscle atrophy caused by stroke or rheumatic diseases. In order to keep muscles under constant motion, during handling, give the muscles a slight twisting force. For rheumatic diseases, however, do not guide the rheumatism factor to the heart.
   b. For muscle injury caused by an acute sprain and moment instant mechanical trauma, dotted and stretched kintape is best to adopt for all injured parts, with relaxation for muscles of injured parts.

As ligaments have no directivity, for ligaments kintape means intensification, but notice that applying kintape to a ligament within joints could cause an adverse reaction that may be different for each individual. For example, applying kintape to the cruciate ligament within the armpit may cause sudden pain (as everyone has a different reaction, it is only used as an example here).

IV. NERVOUS SYSTEM

For the brain and nerve center, generally, apply kintape from nerve endings to terminal. But if there is dotted, tingling pain, apply kintape on the tingling point. If there is continuous numbness and a distension reaction, apply from nerve endings to the direction of the brain, stretching the kintape while applying.

V. MERIDIAN

As I rarely study the meridian system, its cases are not enough to form a unified document and integrated and feasible reaction summary. In practical operation, however, we follow the following purposes or methods:

a. Meridian: take dredging as the main method, reversely apply the kintape according to the trends and direction of movement, i.e. form the flow guidance along with the meridian direction.
b. Reflecting region: according to the reflecting theory of TCM, in the corresponding reflecting region, apply the stretched middle part of the kintape first, and then apply the relaxed both ends of the kintape, to increase the stimulus response of the reflecting region.
c. Acupuncture point: adopt the acupuncture point lifting method to apply. And the purpose is to stimulate the acupuncture point or dredge the acupuncture point.

This aspect still needs to be researched further. It is also expected that additional experts in this aspect should summarize their experiences and operation specifications.

PART II:
PRECAUTIONS FOR OPERATION AND METHOD

1. NOTEWORTHY POINTS DURING THE OPERATION

I. CLEANING
If the skin surface has too much grease or skin care product residue, the adhesive force of the glue to the human body will be reduced, and the protection or treatment effect will also be reduced. Therefore, it is required to ensure the cleanliness and dryness of the skin before applying. If other adhesives or bandages are needed to be used, apply them after the kintape is applied for best ventilation.

II. HAIR
In use, kintape is often applied to parts with excess body hair. In the case of lesser amounts or shorter hair, hair doesn't have a big influence on the effect of the tape, but in the case of thick or long hair, as the kintape itself can not directly contact skin to change tissue fluid and muscle shape under the skin, the hair will seriously influence the effect. Thus, it is suggested to remove/clip excess hair on the area where the kintape will be applied for the best results.

III. RUBBER SURFACE CONTACT
Medical acrylic acid glue is disposable and cannot be reused. During use, the person applying the kintape should not come in direct contact to the glue. If there is too much contact, sweat stains and grease will be left on the rubber surface and influence viscosity. However, the cleanliness of the rubber surface will be influenced, and may cause allergies for some users.

IV. CONTROL OF TENSILE STRENGTH
The control of tensile strength is very important, and previously we discussed the different tensile strengths for different ranges of application. On the one hand, excessive tensile strength can cause adverse effects in the human body. For example, skin may be torn. On the other hand, when the tensile strength is not proper, deckle edges will occur, so the best method for applying the kintape onto

the human body is to apply in a relaxed state at the beginning, then slowly and linearly stretch, and in the end, slowly and linearly relax, and apply the kintape to the skin surface with no tensile strength at the beginning and end.

V. INFLUENCE OF WATER
If there is obvious moisture on the body surface, the moisture must be wiped off, or the application effect will be reduced.

VI. REPEAT PRESS
After the kintape is applied, use hands to press it in again, in order to ensure a firm application.

VII. POSITION
The movement range of the human body in exercise often exceeds the general state, so set the position of the body properly before applying, or the kintape will easily tear in exercise because of incorrect positioning. Therefore position the body so that for all parts, when the skin is stretched totally, the surface area is the maximum. For joints, apply the kintape when the joint curvature angle is at its biggest. If the patient cannot finish one action but can finish that after the kintape is applied, limit the scope of stretching, especially for the knee and elbow joints.

VIII. APPLYING PERIOD
For applying before exercise, the tensile strength is generally 140%. As sweat stains will form on the part of the kintape rubber surface in contact with skin during exercise, it is suggested to remove the kintape immediately after exercise. During recovery after an injury, the tensile strength is generally 120%, and the application time on the human body shall not exceed 2 - 4 days. If the patient has good somatosensory and strong adaptability without any discomfort, the time can be increased to 7 days or above.

Do not apply the kintape on skin wounds. If kintape must be applied, first apply an isolator such as Vaseline to the skin wounds, and use the Vaseline, etc. to isolate the periphery of application points.

IX. CUTTING

The products on the market can be divided into hand-tearing and non-hand-tearing types. For the hand-tearing type, directly use hands to tear the desired shape in vertical and horizontal directions. For the non-hand-tearing type, use scissors to cut the desired shape. For safety purposes, do not let children handle the scissors. The hand-tearing type kintape produced by Changzhou DL Medical & Health Equipment Co., Ltd. can be torn by adults and children (over 4 years old) by way of tearing:

1. For a person who has enough strength: use the thumb and index finger of the left hand and the right hand respectively to pinch both sides of a certain point on the side face of the kintape. Put the fingers and kintape at a 90° right angle. The hand affixing the kintape in place does not move. The other hand pinches the kintape while not moving, then pushes out forward at a 90° right angle.

2. For children, use the strength-control method adopted by the designer: use the teeth to bite one side of the kintape, and use the hand to directly tear it.

X. PEELING OFF

The viscosity of medical acrylic acid glue is high. Forcefully peeling the kintape off will cause pain, so use warm water to soak at first. Then, with one hand pressing the skin, the other hand peels the kintape off at an angle along with the direction of hair. In order to peel the kintape of lumbar vertebra stretched horizontally (one kintape simultaneously includes two clockwise directions of hair) off, tear the kintape into two halves in the middle, and then peel it from the middle to both sides.

2. OPERATION METHODS

Different operation methods have different effects. There are strict method specifications for different symptoms, so even though the finished shapes of taping methods appear to be the same, the methods used are in fact different and for different diseases.

I. HANDLING OF MUSCLE

The flow guidance function of kintape is inborn, therefore, if adopting a different operation method to handle the muscle, the operator themselves must determine the relaxation and intensification. Guiding the flow of tissue fluid under the skin, in the vast majority of cases, is either harmless or beneficial. In some cases, however, a different operation method must be adopted. For example, when the muscle and blood are handled reversely after a stroke, when the muscle injury needs to wrap the pain point, when a certain slice of muscle in exercise needs to relax while the other slice of muscle needs to intensify, or strength transfer between muscles should be completed.

The method to achieve pure muscular relaxation or intensification is: apply one end of the kintape on the skin, then peel the paper off at first, and then stretch the kintape based on the required proportion; directly apply the whole kintape on the skin, applying from the initial point to the terminal point, and then decide the relaxation or intensification based on the direction of the muscle.

As shown in the Fig. below:

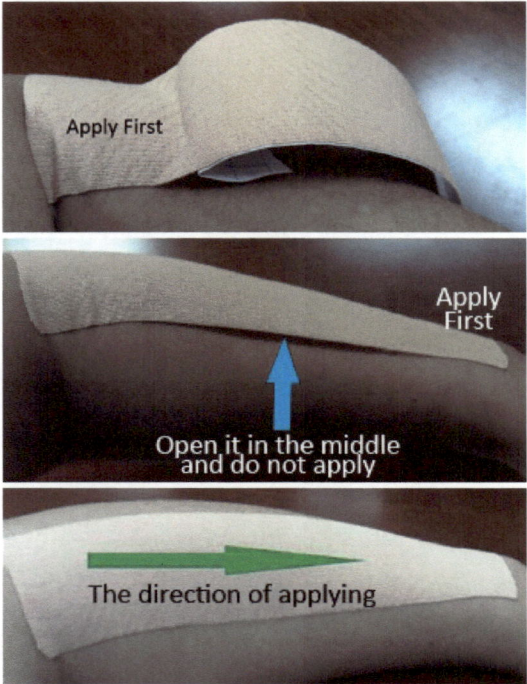

Apply First

Apply First

Open it in the middle and do not apply

The direction of applying

Using this taping method, the kintape has lost the one-way function of creating a venous valve after it covers the skin. The entire force on the skin is not uniformly directing in the same direction, but is exerting force from both sides to the middle of the kintape's entirety. So, the flow guidance function is weakened forcefully, and only handling of the muscle can be finished.

II. HANDLING OF THE TISSUE FLUID

The purpose for handling tissue fluid is to make it flow along the direction according to our requirements, so we must achieve the function of the venous valve. Operation method: apply the initial point of kintape, and apply it while peeling the isolation paper. Both actions shall be finished at the same time. The method can make the kintape form shrink with directivity and form a venous valve with directivity under the skin.

As shown in the Fig. below:

Noteworthy points: for this method, the muscle will be inevitably handled. In some cases, if you do not plan to handle the muscle, you can adopt the following method: 1. Clip the kintape into thin strips, i.e. clip standard kintape with the width of 5 cm into thin strips, such as the width of 1.25 cm. This can minimize its influence on the muscle. 2. Do not apply the kintape on the muscle itself, but apply it on the part between the two slices of the muscle, such as the part between the scapula muscle and the rhomboid muscle or the part between the soleus muscle and the gastrocnemius muscle.

III. HANDLING OF THE SPACE UNDER THE SKIN

The purpose for handling the space under the skin is to lift the skin, and stretch the adhesion of the muscle and skin to achieve the function of dredging, and provide further flow guidance with space. There are two methods of handling: One method is to relax the middle part of the kintape and stretch the periphery of both sides when applying. Thus, the peripheral skin is intensified, while the skin of the middle part is relaxed and lifted (Fig. I below). The other one is to stretch the middle part and relax the periphery or both sides to apply (Fig. II below). Therefore, as kintape is gathered into the middle part, the middle part will be lifted directly, such as the handling of the temple. Make different judgments based on different situations to use these two techniques. The main factors that shall be considered are their influences on the peripheral skin and muscles. For example, use the first technique to handle lumbar vertebra (as lumbar vertebra is dented, a flat application to the surrounding skin can lift the skin in the middle. Meanwhile, the relaxed application in the middle part can prevent the kintape from leaving the skin).

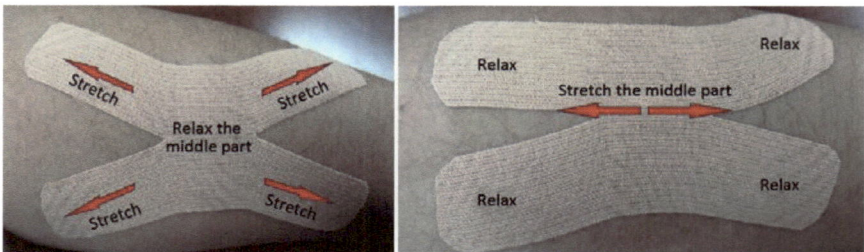

Fig. I

IV. HANDLING OF NERVES AND ACUPUNCTURE POINTS

The purpose for handling nerves and acupuncture points is to stimulate the nerves and achieve a dredging function. Therefore, the handling method is to intensify the touch input on the handling point, increase the pressure to acupuncture points, or stretch more on the handling point while stretching less on the adjacent position.

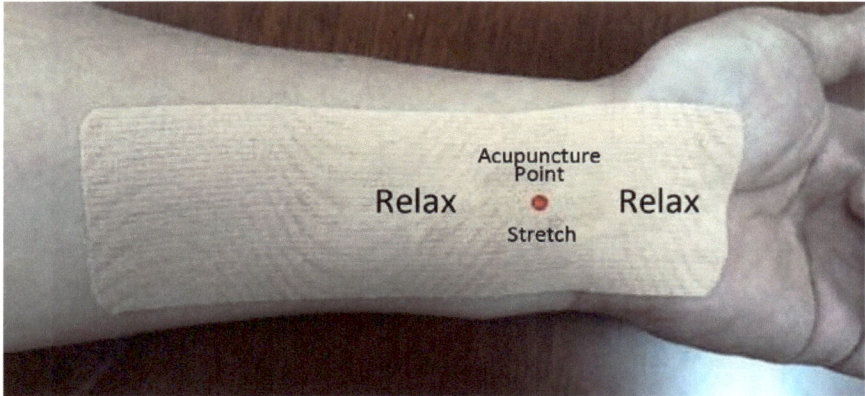

Fig. II

V. HANDLING OF STRENGTH TRANSFER

After an injury, if rest is required for the muscle of a certain part to make the injury recover as soon as possible, or to limit pressure on the injury while maintaining normal function of the body part, and to minimize the influence of the injury on exercising the part to a great extent, strength in the exercise must be transferred to another relevant muscle group, so strength transfer is necessary. Operation method: apply the stretched kintape on the injured part, and then conduct relaxation handling on the injured muscle group (pay attention to the blood flow direction), reversely handle the muscle group that needs to transfer strength, and intensify strength. For the method of this part, refer to the handling method of the muscle.

Strength transfer here is to realize different functions on the same kintape, but not to realize different functions by many.

See Fig. III for operation instructions.

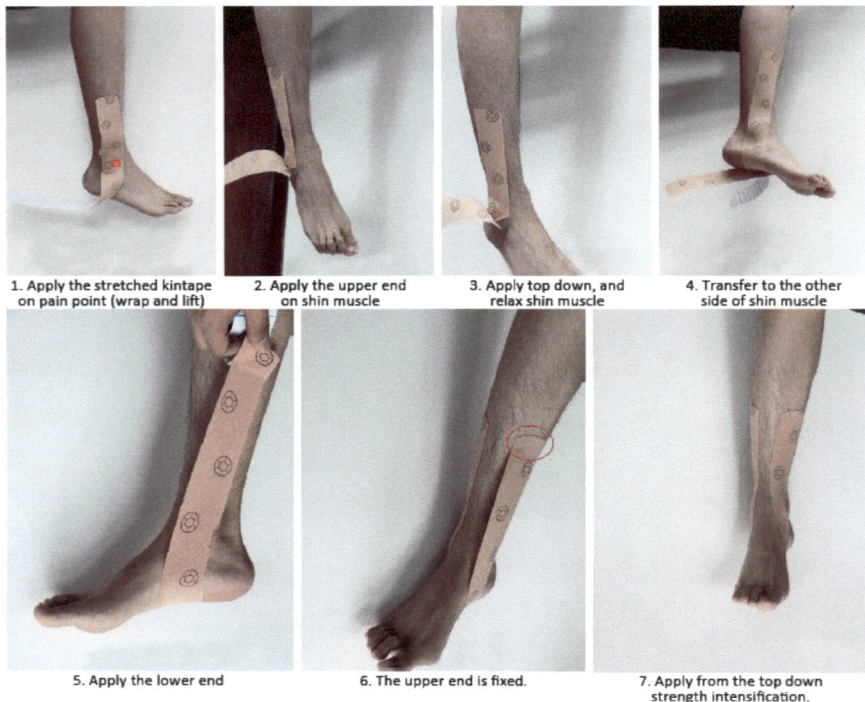

| 1. Apply the stretched kintape on pain point (wrap and lift) | 2. Apply the upper end on shin muscle | 3. Apply top down, and relax shin muscle | 4. Transfer to the other side of shin muscle |

| 5. Apply the lower end | 6. The upper end is fixed. | 7. Apply from the top down strength intensification. |

Fig. III

VI. CONTROL OF TENSILE STRENGTH

The control of tensile strength directly refers to the application scope and purpose. When using for treatment, do not stretch the kintape excessively for an instantaneous feeling. The control degree shall be 120%, 140% for sports and 160% for first-aid types. Products provided by Changzhou DL Medical & Health Equipment Co., Ltd. can be controlled through little soccer balls printed on the surface or weaved graphic change. When the control degree reaches 120%, the control can be realized by peeling the release paper off directly and utilizing the release force of paper. During the application, however, the following circumstances are not limited:

1. When disposing one point on the whole bar, the stretching range can be increased. If there are different strength requirements, users can realize different tensile strengths in one bar, even various different values may arise, as shown in Fig. IV.

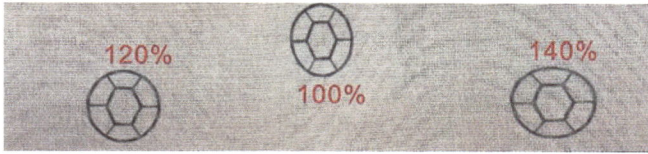

Fig. IV

2. When using the kintape in a small area, users can stretch it fully, which is unrelated to the first-aid application. For example, for analgesia of impact injury in one point, or angiectasis in the temple.

VII. FORMATION OF PRESSURE DIFFERENCES

When applying striping types (such as Y or claw type) of kintape, if the flow guidance technique is adopted, since it is impossible to apply the same force and tensile strength to each bar, the backflow speed on each branch will be different. When coming together at one point, the pressure difference will take shape between different branches on the same kintape, and will promote the circulation of subcutaneous tissue fluid. In some circumstances, it will promote the healing of symptoms. These shall be taken into consideration during actual operations. In some applications, it may be valuable. For example, not only the flow guidance, but also right and left pressure differences will take shape on the musculus biceps brachii of stroke patients. This will intensify the tension state of muscle and make for recovery. If branches are not in different sizes, different pressure differences will take shape, as shown in the Fig. below. When the same two branches are applied onto the same muscle or position, as in the abovementioned principle, the pressure difference will take shape as well.

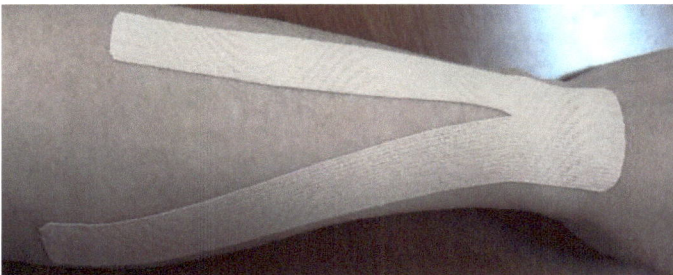

Different tensile strengths form pressure differences
Flow guidance rate is different

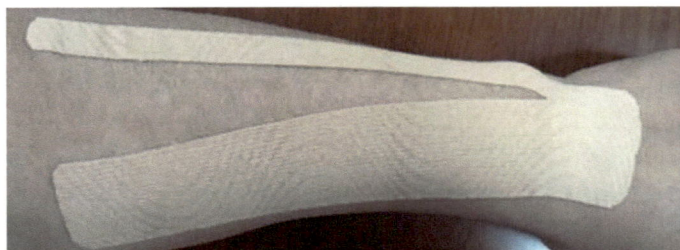

Different bar widths form different pressure differences

Due to the difference in techniques of operators and symptoms in specific circumstances, other application methods are to be further perfected and summarized by researchers and users in actual operation.

3. COMMON SHAPES AND BASIC EFFECTS

Different shapes of kintapes have different functions. To achieve these functions, different shapes shall be combined. Here, a brief introduction and discussion of the basic effects of common shapes is provided.

Common clipping figures can generally be classified into five types, i.e. I, Y, X and O type as well as a dispersing type (the previously mentioned claw type). The dispersing type can be further classified into one-end dispersing and middle dispersing types. Description of the effects and the usage of five common figures is as follows:

I. I TYPE

This type is also called vertical-bar type. Applying different directions of force can both relax and contract the muscle. The results of stretching and taping methods are as follows, respectively:

a. First, stretch and apply it at one end, then stretch the kintape evenly and apply it onto the skin while stretching. Applying in different directions of the muscle can relax or enhance the muscle strength in the applied position. Meanwhile, it has the effect of one-way flow guidance. For the results of the effect, the tensile strength is in direct proportion to the capacity of the flow guidance and muscle treatment. It is of the strongest ability in flow guidance among all forms.

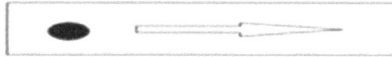

b. First, apply the kintape in the middle point, then stretch at both ends and apply it onto the skin while it is stretched. It can make the skin at two ends approach toward the middle and converge toward one point. This can support the injured position by enhancing the muscular strength around it. At this time, it has obvious effects on opening the subcutaneous space, but effects of the flow guidance are weakened and it has no obvious effects on changes in the muscular strength.

c. First, stretch it at two ends. When it is fully stretched, apply both ends on the smooth skin surface. Then, apply the rest onto the skin in order to make the covered skin produce wrinkles and relax the muscle evenly, producing no tensile force or flow force in a single-point direction. When the I-type kintape is in a wrapped form, this method will fix and massage the sore spot. At this moment, it will change the muscular strength in a limited range while changing the skin's touch significantly and lifting the whole skin.

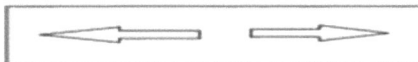

d. First, stretch it at one end and apply the end onto the initial point, then stretch it fully and apply it onto another point. Finally apply the rest, pressing toward the terminal point from the initial point, or toward the initial point from the terminal point. At this moment, its main effects are strengthening or relaxing the muscle. However, the effects of flow guidance and skin lifting are weakened.

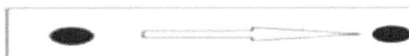

II. Y TYPE

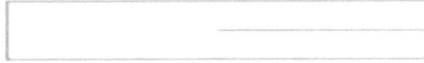

Also called one-end bifurcated type, it can wrap muscle groups. Based on different force bearing points, it also has the effect of support pulling, one-way retraction, surface skin lifting, muscle relaxation or strengthening, as well as the formation of right and left pressure differences. Corresponding instructions are as follows:

a. First, apply the connection points, stretch the bifurcations and wrap the muscle groups in circularity to fix wrapped muscle groups. The central point retracts inward, and directions of flow guidance gather toward connection points. When muscle groups are wrapped in circularity, the pressure difference takes shape between these two branches. Iit can be generally applied right above the area of the muscle to make the muscle proceed to a locomotive state.

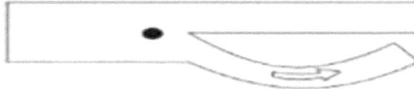

b. First, affix the connection points, then two bifurcations shall be applied onto the skin while stretching evenly. This will make the skin form the venous valve effects of flowing to joint points. When applying in an opposite direction of muscle, it will relax the muscle and slow down the blood backflow. When applying in the same direction of muscle, it will strengthen the muscular strength and promote the improvement of blood oxygen content. The connection points are usually applied near lymph glands (when it is ascertained to be a non-bacterial inflammation). Bifurcated branches are usually applied onto the joints of the two adjacent muscle groups to treat fascia tissue fluid at joints. It is generally used in clearing non-bacterial inflammation.

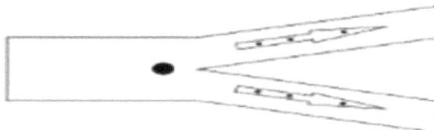

c. First, apply the joint points, then stretch the bifurcated branches' entirety and apply it onto the skin surface flatly. Since the force of connection points may not comply with that of bifurcated branches, lifting may take shape underneath the skin in joint points or bifurcated branches. Open the subcutaneous space and the skin retracts in one direction. Meanwhile, treat the skin beneath the bifurcated branches. However, the force as well as effects and the speed of flow guidance in this type are inferior to that of I type (vertical-bar type). In addition, the coverage is larger than other types.

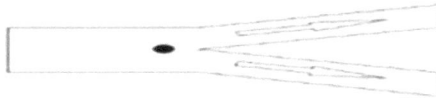

d. First apply bifurcations, stretch it in an arc or straight direction and apply it onto the middle part. Then apply it onto the joint points to support the muscle and cause larger areas of muscle in the joint points to shrink upward. Using different exerting ways, meanwhile, can form a reacting force, two forces that will act on the central bifurcation point to form a triangular wear-stress zone. Muscles in the zone will be forcefully supported. For this technique, it is usually very difficult to achieve flow guidance since the operation technique is harder.

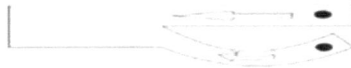

III. X TYPE

It is also called cross type. Its main effects are increasing the circulation of blood or tissue fluid in the applied position, as well as lifting the skin of sore spots. When used separately, it can be used directly as an analgesic plaster. When combined with other shapes, it is mostly used to prepare for the next step or shape. In combined sets, therefore, it is the first shape to be applied. The main taping methods are:

    a. Apply the central point onto the sore spot, stretch and apply the four branches in four directions to form a skin shrinkage effect toward the middle sore spot. It is the equivalent of a massage for the sore spot. Meanwhile, it may stretch the skin around the sore spot reversely in four directions. As a result, the skin in the middle is lifted and the subcutaneous space is opened.

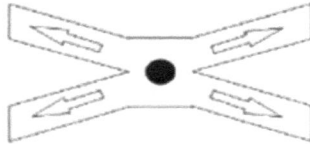

    b. First, stretch the four corners and apply onto the skin surface directly, then affix the middle point at the sore spot or a point that requires treatment to tighten wrinkles toward the skin in the middle. It will promote the blood circulation of subcutaneous tissue. The whole applied surface is lifted and has a certain degree of warp. When the muscle skin is stiff, the effect of flow guidance is not obvious while the pain is relieved. When the skin is loose, wrinkles increase and the inward tightening effects are better.

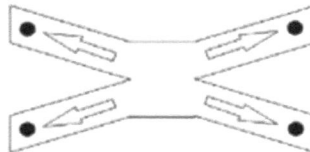

    c. First, stretch and apply the middle part, then apply the four corners naturally. The lifting height of the middle position in this way is higher than that of the taping method in (a), while the surrounding somatic sense is inferior to that in (a). It is usually applicable to positions requiring intense lifting, such as blood balance in the case of migraine seizures and acute treatment in the case of Achilles ruptures. The intensity degree is excessive in treating chronic common diseases.

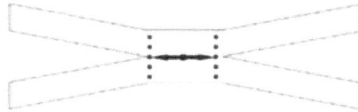

IV. O TYPE

It is also called the middle strip-cutting type, and is mainly used to fix and massage injured positions and form stability in the location to be treated. It is seldom used. However, it can be used when the injured position is difficult to treat and no flow guidance is expected, when a relatively closed pressure difference should be formed.

a. First, stretch it lengthways and affix the two ends. Stretch and apply the two strips bifurcated in the middle to form the pressing force toward the middle as a massage. Meanwhile, it will fix the form of the delineated range, and lift the whole delineated muscles and skin. No flow guidance will be formed in the circle and under the kintape to be applied.

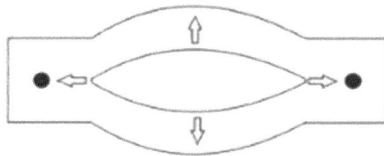

b. First, apply the two bifurcations, then stretch the two ends toward both sides and apply it onto the skin surface to form an inward convergent force from both sides. Meanwhile, the two ends also have the force to converge toward the two pre-fixed points. The surface skin in the pre-applied points will be lifted and the flow guidance moves toward the two pre-applied points (side edging).

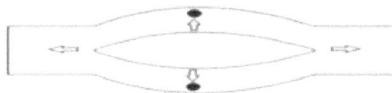

V. DISPERSING TYPE

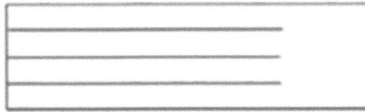

It is also called claw type, and is generally used to treat silting and expansion, lumps, and create flow guidance as well as realign subcutaneous fascia.

a. First, apply the connection points, then apply the claw branches while stretching. Take flow guidance as the principal and the fixed point as the final trend point. It is generally used in detumescence, swelling as well as varicosity. Claw branches are usually covering swelling points, with fixed points connected near the heart end. When being applied in varicosity, apply branches in the varicosity positions requiring treatment, and apply the connected ends near the blood return point of the venous blood vessels. If rigescent (stiff or numb) muscle is needed, it is in general the most common shape, applied along the direction of the muscle (enhancement) or blood vessel backflow.

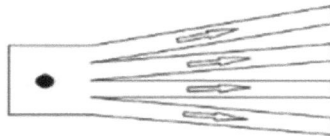

b. When two claw kintapes are applied in a cross with a certain angle while the fixed end is close to the heart position (common position, not necessarily the case - other crosses are allowed with weakened effects), the blood pressure at the cross site will be forced to break, and the blood circulation will be accelerated violently and expand continuously. In the end, the entirety of the involved blood system is much higher in pressure than the area to be applied. For detumescence and the treatment of varicosity, if applicable, treat these two simultaneously. It shall be noted that a single bar has the function of one-way flow guidance. And when two or more bars are used together, it is not one-way flow guidance but a circulatory system instead.

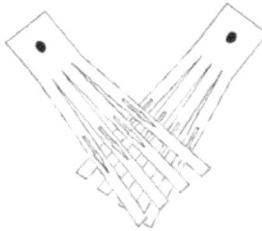

c. Sort out the fascia to diffuse extravasated blood. Apply dispersion points one after another. Then stretch branches while applying until reaching the connection points, to form a force direction toward dispersion points and guide the flow from one point to the bifurcations. This is generally applied to clear extravasated blood in one point, or when flow directions of the blood and lymph contradict with that of muscles, germs, etc. in treating problems involving blood, lymph, etc.

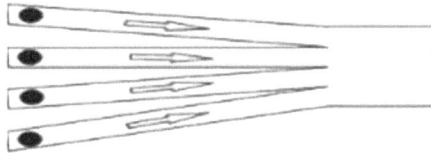

d. Combine two claw kintapes, i.e., connected in the middle and divided into claw type at two ends. For this taping method, first apply the middle section and then apply the branches while stretching to achieve the exchange of energy and substance in the middle point (acupuncture points effect). For application, the interposition is usually applied onto the injured point. Two claw kintapes are separately for lymph or blood. The applied position in the middle will be lifted as well. The effects are inferior to that of X type or other shapes while the effects of flow guidance and exchange are optimum. Particular circumstances, such as swelling and other potential inflammation, will cause the claw kintape on one side to cover the swelling position as well; the claw kintape on the other side will try to collect the blood or lymph. The middle section lies between the two points, corresponding to a treatment center.

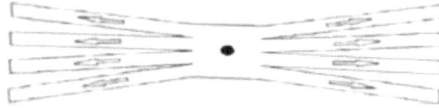

Considerations for all the above applications:

1. The starts of all kintapes shall not be stretched and must be completely tension-free;
2. There shall be a buffer between the tension-free site and the stretched site to avoid sudden change (cliff-type cutting);
3. All ends must be tension-free;
4. The tension-free front section and tension-free rear section at all ends shall form a buffer to avoid sudden change (cliff-type cutting);
5. The tensile strength is overall subject to the specification of 120%, 140%, and 160% while tapering range and special applications are not.

4. SOME FACTORS INFLUENCING FINAL EFFECTS

First, we need to affirm that kintape is not all-purpose. We can understand the operator's attitude of making it better, and that good usage will help patients relieve the pain, but the kintape is essentially a physical therapy, realizing its functions by coinciding with and guiding the functions of the human body. It is not capable of affecting internal tissue of the human body for change, unlike chemical agents.

Since it is merely a physical therapy, and dedicated medical equipment will not be used for earlier diagnosis in many circumstances, the first factor influencing the final effect of kintape application is diagnosis.

The first key point for judgment: is it a bacterial inflammation? If yes, we recommend other ways to be used for treatment since we are not sure whether this type of inflammation will damage the lymph, and we shall not waste the optimum treatment time of consumers. A distinct case is infection caused by the cold virus that results in a skin injury. It cannot be treated with kintape. Another distinct case is quinsy, as it may be a viral or bacterial inflammation. For types of inflammation that cannot be judged, users will need to avoid the introduction of inflammation into lymph glands when introducing lymph into focus points during operation.

The second key point for judgment: injury causes, such as treating scapulohumeral periarthritis as a frozen shoulder. The success of treatment is directly related to the knowledge of what is causing the injury, as well as which parts are affected. For example, with ankle pain, it may be an injury from a collision or sprain, myotenositis, or even an old wound. There can be no successful treatment unless the cause is judged accurately.

The third key point for judgment: feelings of the patient, soreness, anaesthesia, pain, expansion. and other sensations. They usually represent different causes and treatment programs. In many cases, different feelings may interlace. According to my experience, the common judgment principle for frequently appearing feelings or sensations is as follows, it shall be noted that the principle is not absolutely correct.

Limp: generally caused by a lack of muscle strength or excessive fatigue. When a strength deficiency, apply the methods of strengthening or increasing blood oxygen content. When the cause is excessive fatigue, apply the methods of relaxing and accelerating blood circulation. If it is relatively severe, further apply the method of lymph import.

Numb: it is generally obstruction of the blood or nerves. Usual treatment consists of applying the methods of reversely suppressing the blood flow rate or relaxing the oppressed or constricted nerve bundle.

Sore: soreness generally results from injuries that have occurred and, at many times, inflammation will occur synchronously. Sometimes, muscle or ligament has been torn. The common method is to shrink and fix the sore spot. Treat the subcutaneous space, and create blood circulation and flow guidance in the case of swelling. Increase strength transition if the injured point must withstand strength.

If the pain is throughout the whole body and is present when touching, there is a higher probability of occurrence at the back. Treatment of blood circulation for the whole back if indicated, generally with positive effects.

Swelling: it mainly occurs in the four limbs. It may be caused by injury of a muscle or tendon, or by the non-circulation of blood. In most cases, use the blood circulation or flow guidance methods. If swelling occurs due to bone injury, it cannot be treated by kintape. Seek medical treatment as soon as possible.

The second factor that can affect the final effect of kintape application is the individuality of patients. Different symptoms and taping methods on different human bodies will cause different reactions. For example, for knee pain, the knee may feel either hot or cold depending on the temperature of the person in question. If the body is overheated, the knee will generally feel hot. If the person is cool, the pain may present with coldness. Treatment method and application must be according to individual differences. For another example, with lumbar muscle strain where the application of kintape downwards exceeds the Zhi Shi acupoint (lumbar eye), if the person applied is an athlete, there are no adverse reactions, but if the person applied is a normal office worker, he/she may feel limp. If the person applied is a relatively weak elder, there may be no reaction.

The third factor: the understanding of kintape by the operator. We have discussed previously that there are very few people who know about kintape, and there are still less people that know about its basic principles. For the people I contacted, they just kept trying and summarizing reactions of a certain symptom with different methods. Due to not understanding the principles and operational norms of kintape, they are not able to correctly anticipate the results after being applied. The reason for the current situation is mainly due to the split of production and research of kintape worldwide, i.e. users or researchers don't know how kintape is produced or its standards and requirements, while producers don't know how kintape is used. They are the equivalent of two parallel lines and cannot find a breakthrough point of convergence into the other side. This is one of the reasons that I am writing and publishing this book, to further expand knowledge and practical use with operators, researchers, and manufacturers.

The fourth factor: the product itself. Using the same taping method, with the same person and the same symptom, if products of different brands or manufacturers are used you will find the results are sometimes effective and sometimes ineffective. It is because the product manufacturing standards are different according to different manufacturers. Many projects are similar in form or appearance without being similar in function.

The fifth factor: operating method. For the operating method, knowing what we are trying to accomplish and how is of primary importance. Without meaning to, many operators make basic errors even with common applications. As far as I know, there are no training agencies and manufacturers yet that really specify the operating method required. For example, an injury obviously requires muscle relaxation, but flow guidance is done. In addition, operating methods are divided into categories such as lifting and depressing, lightly or heavily, pulling and withdrawing. The error cannot be seen simply from the applied shape.

The sixth factor: associated elements are inadequately considered. This is a phenomenon that has occurred many times. For example, the nervous system is taken into account but the influence to the blood is not considered. Or the relaxation of muscles in taken into account but the blood of the muscle is cut off. A third example is when the intensification of the muscle is taken into account but the next muscle group is negatively affected due to extending the kintape 1 cm more, etc.

The seventh factor: weather or external elements. Under the same condition, the blood flow rate of the human body will be slower in winter than in summer. Soreness and a sense of powerlessness are easier to generate on rainy days. In operation, if this is not taken into consideration and appropriate adjustments aren't made, the final effect will be influenced.

The eighth factor: self-change of the disease or injury. The same disease, through the suitable treatment mentioned above, will be better. However, another reaction that is originally hidden may occur. If that happens, the operator must make appropriate adjustments so as to generate a beneficial effect. Otherwise, the final effect will be influenced. For example, the first symptom for patients with cervical spondylopathy is soreness in the neck and stiffness of the shoulder. After a period of relaxation and subcutaneous opening up, this symptom is definitely better, but patients may feel discomfort at their back. And some patients may now notice that the neck now has a soreness in the semispinalis muscles. Actually, these problems existed originally. It is just that at the beginning, symptoms of soreness in the neck and stiffness in the shoulder are more obvious, and patients fail to experience the other secondary sore parts or don't deem them as the primary problems to be settled. When the primary problems are settled, the operator must make the appropriate adjustments to settle the secondary problems. In another example, the initial patients with a frozen shoulder all exhibit the following symptoms: a certain point around the shoulder is sore and sometimes may have a sense of cold pain. Additional symptoms such as an inability to raise the arms, or rotate inward or outward will occur. However, after several kintape applications, deep muscle pain about 1 cm under the shoulder will occur. In fact, this is blood loss in the surface caused by the treatment of deep pain, and it will cause a mild injury to the muscle. This is inevitable, but the focal point of work by the operator shall be adjusted to treat these sore muscles.

The ninth factor: patient problems. We have mentioned before that kintape is not a universal solution and that many diseases cannot be treated through it. However, even when treating an injury or disease that can be affected by kintape, there can be additional problems, such as discovering a severe skin allergy to the glue, which would generate an adverse reaction. Another situation is if the patient has additional medical issues that need to be taken into consideration. For example, when treating a headache, if the patient has hypotension, standard taping methods will have no effect or may even cause dizziness. In another example, I had treated a case where the patient's legs were severely swollen and were so sore that he couldn't rest. Through three courses of treatment, the pain relief effect decreased first from 4 hours to 2 hours, and then after the third treatment, he felt sore even immediately after the kintape was applied. It had puzzled me for quite a long time. Later, I learned that the patient had leukemia and the pain was caused by the disease. His family hid the condition from him. Without knowing these additional circumstances, I was unable to adjust the taping methods, and the kintape had no effect on his pain.

The elements mentioned above cannot incorporate all the factors that influence the final effect, though it is a good start. Hopefully more researchers will summarize and make the use of kintape, allowing more normalization and standardization as well as insight into additional factors that change how kintape is used.

CHAPTER IV: COMMON ADVERSE REACTIONS AND CAUSES

In the process of using kintape, operators and users will find many adverse reactions, including issues with the product itself and adverse reactions generated in the users' bodies. Detailed descriptions are accordingly set as below:

I. COMMON REACTIONS CAUSED BY THE PRODUCT ITSELF

1. THE KINTAPE FALLS OFF OR SLIPS SEVERAL MINUTES AFTER BEING APPLIED.
   a. Generally, it takes about 15 min for the glue to solidify. Before the glue is totally solidified, it is easy to peel, and it will seem that the viscosity is inadequate. Doing substantial movements at this time will cause the tension of the kintape to be larger than the cohesive force with the skin, which can cause the kintape to droop, slide, or even fall off. The solution is to give a sufficient solidification time to the glue.
   b. It is not applied firm and there is part of the tape not connected to the skin. The solution is to press the kintape with a hand in the direction of application to ensure that the kintape has been fully tightened with the skin, or that the upper layer and the lower layer of the adhesive tapes have been fully tightened with each other.
   c. The medical propenoic acid glue is disposable glue and after being fully applied and solidified, it can be waterproof and

sweatproof. But if there is water or sweat on the body when applying, the viscosity of the glue will be significantly reduced. The solution is to wipe off the sweat with a napkin or towel and blow it dry as appropriate, making the solidification time longer.

2. THE ENDS/EDGES OF THE KINTAPE ARE ROLLING/FLANGING.
   a. This is generated by the constant friction of the clothing, which will make the kintape peel. The solution is to wear relatively loose clothes or clothes that fit well with the surface of the body.
   b. The stretched length of the adhesive tape is too long when applying, or the superficial area of the skin does not fit maximally. So, in body movement, the complete stretched length of the adhesive tape is inadequate and will cause it to roll up. The solution is to: 1. Reduce the stretched length when applying. 2. Change the posture of the patient when applying to make it possible to increase the superficial area of the skin.
   c. If the ends of the kintape are stretched when applying, or if the stretched length is too large, the internal stress of the reverse contraction of the kintape is too great. The contraction force at the complete extension of the skin is larger than the cohesive force, so it can cause the edges to peel and roll. The solution is to reduce the tension at the beginning and the end when applying kintape.

3. IT SEEMS GOOD AT THE BEGINNING AFTER BEING APPLIED, BUT FEELS SORE LATER.
   a. If the length of the kintape is too long, it can affect more than one muscle group. For example, if one kintape is applied to a muscle to intensify that area of the muscle , but one end of the kintape is applied to another area of the muscle, it generates relaxation to the other area of the muscle. The opposite it true if generating relaxation and accidentally causing intensification in another muscle group. The solution is to tear up or cut away the redundant kintape on the other area of the muscle. When distinguishing the muscle, users can see from the external

features of the muscle that there is an obvious joint (muscle sag) at the boundary of the two muscles.

b. The direction is opposite. It conducts relaxation when aimed at intensification. The solution is to re-apply it in the opposite direction (replace the kintape).

c. When applying claw types, one or more claw types cut off the main and collateral channels. The solution is to sort out the directions of the branches of claw types, and not to cut off one of the main and collateral channels. It is the same for blood circulation.

d. When wrapping laterally, the distortional deformation is generated in two or more muscle groups laterally, making the distortional muscle in tension status and causing soreness. The solution is to:

    i.   remove the lateral wrapping;

    ii. pull open the middle of the kintape and then apply toward the two sides.

4. THE LIMBS CLOSE TO THE END ARE SWELLED.

If applied at the part near joints, the laterally applied kintape could have too large an inward pressure that presses on the veins and causes the blood at the body surface not to reflow to the heart. The solution is to remove the laterally applying kintape or change it to the diagonal taping method (U-type taping method).

5. IT STARTS OUT HELPING BUT THERE IS PAIN WHEN EXERCISING.

a. Excessive exercise can exceed the limit of physical performance. The solution is to stop exercising and rest.

b. The muscle is strengthened again with a second application of kintape during exercise, but the direction or taping method of the added kintape conflicts with that of the former one. The solution is to remove the added kintape, and if the muscle needs to strengthened again, add a second application based on the former one, or apply close to the former one along with its direction.

II. REACTIONS DURING TREATMENT AND RECOVERY

1. ITCH
   a. The kintape is stretched too much when applying, causing the speed of flow guidance to exceed that of the blood circulation that can be borne by the subcutaneous space. Generally, it is generated at the edge of the kintape or at the two ends of the kintape. Sometimes, it is because of the excessive stimulation to the skin by the kintape. The solution is to stretch the kintape with the principle of not exceeding 120% of the original length (with paper). For our products, please see the pattern printed at the surface of the kintape. To reach 120% stretch, just pull the oval outside to a circle.
   b. The fascia space blocked subcutaneously is opened and the tissue fluid flows according to the direction of applying, which conflicts with the original stationary state. The solution is to apply several times, creating a habitual flow.
   c. Failure of adaptation by the skin. The solution is to softly pull the kintape when starting the application. Give the skin time to adapt to the kintape and slowly increase the pulling length.
   d. If the itch is at the outermost end of the kintape: if the kintape exerts a downward stress to the skin at the starting and ending parts of the application, and the blood is relatively blocked at the junction, this causes blood accumulation, leading to the itchy sensation. The solution is to: 1. Uncover the kintape a little at the itchy part and remove it. 2. Wholly uncover the kintape at the itchy part and apply on it again, or cut it off. 3. Apply the starting and ending parts under a fully relaxed status.

2. ITCH WITH VESICLES
   a. The strength of the stretched kintape is too great and corrugation occurs on the skin under the applied tape. The solution is to remove the tape until the skin recovers. When applying the next time: first, the strength (of the stretch) must be lessened. Second, the applied skin must be wholly flat to avoid creating corrugation under the kintape.
   b. The speed of flow guidance is too fast and the subcutaneous

space cannot afford it, generating an accumulated point at the junction and causing blood blisters. Generally, according to the direction of the applying, the blister at the starting point is inside the kintape, while the one at the other side is outside the kintape. In some conditions, the same situation will occur in the vertical edge of the kintape. The solution is to stretch as slow as possible at the beginning and then speed up until the subcutaneous space slowly expands. Both the starting and ending parts shall be applied in a fully relaxed state to form a slow transition from the pulling open/stretched part.

c. Chill in the body of the applied patient is too much, causing cold to be exported from the joints. The surface phenomenon of blisters occurs, and sometimes it may be slightly yellow.

3. THERE NOTHING WHEN APPLYING AT THE WAIST BUT A SORE FEELING WHEN APPLYING AT THE BOTTOM.
The kintape exceeds the waist line (Zhi Shi acupoint) when making a strip down (or slashing down) the waist.

The solution is to:
a. Try to endure it if it must be done so.
b. Directly strip off the excessive part and the soreness will disappear immediately.
c. Change the direction when applying the strip, e.g. change from top-down to inside-out.
d. The applied part isn't painful but other parts are. In fact, other parts may be sore, but the more painful part conceals the soreness at this part. When the soreness at other parts is treated, the soreness at this part will be transferred to the nerve. The solution is to treat the latter soreness.

III. BODY PARTS WITH VARIOUS SYMPTOMS IN COMMON DISEASES/INJURIES

1. MEDIAL KNEE JOINT NEAR SHANK

Symptoms: Itch at the front end of the tape and slight redness after being stripped.

Cause: Pulling too much at the beginning. Apply the start of the kintape in a fully relaxed status. If it occurs continuously, it is because after being fully relaxed at the beginning, the ratio difference of the pulling force generated at the latter part and the strength at the part under fully relaxed status is too great.

Solution: a. Strip off the front end of the tape and cut it off.
b. After the start of the kintape is applied well, slowly stretch the kintape as applying to the skin and don't pull it abruptly.
c. Move up the starting point of the kintape application.

2. SHOULDER NEAR JIANJING ACUPOINT

Symptoms: Itchy and sore with a skin-tearing sensation, especially after a shower.

Cause: The force pulling toward the back is too great.

Solution: a. Cut the tape longer to exceed the shoulder and apply under a fully relaxed status.
b. The pulling open/stretched elasticity should be smaller.

3. WAIST

Symptoms: Extremely unbearable itch.

Cause: The waist muscle and subcutaneous space have been rigid and are now forced to be open and activated.

Solution: a. Softly stretch the kintape when beginning to apply, and add strength appropriately with the increasing time of applying to give the subcutaneous space time to expand.
b. Don't use tape the first time. Use vitality cream to relax the subcutaneous, repeat for several times, and then apply.

4. SHOULDER

Symptoms: The most painful part of the frozen shoulder feels itchy. The principle is the same with that of the waist.

Symptoms: The shoulder moves freely but under the surface it feels very painful (especially when touched).

Cause: The inflammation inside the shoulder is extracted to the surface. The soreness at the deep layer is transferred to the surface.

Solution: The solution is to direct the flow guidance to the lymph. (Note: such symptoms occur in at least 4 out of 5 times of effective applications.)

5. KNEE

Symptoms: The top of the patella feels itchy.

Cause: Since the blood at the top is guided to the armpits and generates a large amount of circulation, the originally cold and rigid patella top cannot adapt to it at once.

Solution: a. Stretch the claw kintape as softly and gently as possible when applying.
b. Touch and stroke it with the hand.

Symptoms: It doesn't feel itchy until the tape is stripped off.

Cause: The circulation channel doesn't form regularity and the blood flows according to its original patterns after the kintape is stripped off.

Solution: Apply continuously until a regular and habitual operational circulation is formed.

Symptoms: Itch with vesicles.

Cause: a. the stretched force is too great;
b. is there rheumatism?
c. Corrugation on the skin.

Solution: a. the strength shall be as soft as possible.
b. Apply until the vesicles of rheumatism or rheumatoid arthritis break, and rub some cool cream.
c. Stroke until the skin is flat (especially for an elder).

6. MEDIAL AND LATERAL THIGH

Symptoms: Itch with skin damage.

Cause: Kintape is pulled too much at the beginning.

Solution: Apply at the beginning with the length under fully relaxed status of more than 4 cm to reduce the displacement generated on the skin.

IV. WITH NO EFFECT OR THE EFFECT NOT BEING OBVIOUS

First, for symptoms that the kintape can treat, it is generally effective if judged suitably and applied using the qualified operating method and products. However, taking consideration of the body constitution of the patient themselves, the reaction period may sustain for 1 or 2 days.

CHAPTER V: PRACTICAL TAPING TECHNIQUES

I. HEADACHE

1. CAUSE OF DISEASE
    a. Cervical vertebra;
    b. Hyperpiesia or hypotension;
    c. Vascular sclerosis or inhibited blood reflow.

2. SYMPTOMS
    a. Dizziness or headache;
    b. Dazzle and difficulty standing or walking;
    c. Blood vessel breakout;
    d. Canthus turns red.

3. TAPING METHOD FIG. AND TECHNIQUE DESCRIPTION

THE FIRST KINTAPE
Pull open the middle part and apply.
Apply on the Temple acupoint and relax at the two ends.

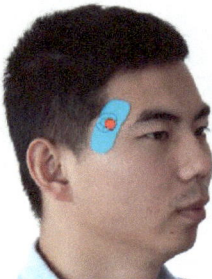

THE SECOND KINTAPE
The same method
Apply on the Temple acupoint on the other side.
See Fig. after completing the first and the second kintapes.

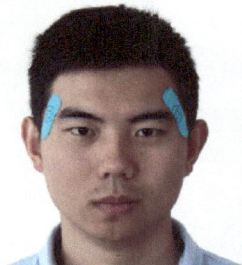

THE THIRD KINTAPE
Apply down along shoulder to neck, and directly pull the paper without pulling the fabrics.

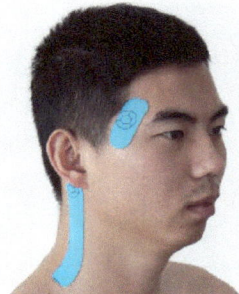

TECHNIQUE DESCRIPTION

The first and second kintapes are stretched at the middle part, and the two ends are applied under a relaxed state. The purpose is to enhance the subcutaneous space at the Temple acupoint and expand the blood vessel at the trigeminus.

The third kintape is stretched and applied from shoulder to neck. The operating method is flow guidance. The part is chosen at the venous return point near the neck. The purpose is to conduct the flow guidance of blood in the head to the heart to achieve balance of the blood pressure in the head.

4. REACTIONS AFTER APPLYING

For symptoms: hypertension, migraine, balance damage of blood pressure in the head due to drinking, or other causes. The Temple acupoint feels cool after it is applied and the head feels clear. The headache will reduce in about 5 minutes. It if is caused by hypertension, the blood pressure in the head reduces when measuring the blood pressure.

5. NOTE:
   a. It is prohibited to apply like this for hypotension.
   b. The third kintape cannot be applied oppositely no matter what the situation.

II. CERVICAL SPONDYLOPATHY

1. CAUSE OF DISEASE
   a. Cervical intervertebral disc degeneration and water content decrease, inducing or promoting tissue metamorphosis in other positions;
   b. Keeping the same posture for a long time produces muscle and ligament fatigue;
   c. Throat infection, wind-cold-dampness invasion, long-term poor mood, fatigue, etc.

2. SYMPTOMS

a. Early symptoms are aches in the neck, shoulder, and arm, stiffness in neck, and limited movement;

b. Keeping a fixed posture for a long time produces pain, swelling, and stiffness in the nape. Aches in the neck and shoulder may be extended to occipital region and upper limbs;

c. Sometimes it is accompanied by dizziness, i.e., the room revolving. In patients with severe conditions, it may be accompanied by nausea and vomiting, while some may be accompanied by vertigo and cataplexy;

d. In patients with severe conditions it may be accompanied by a sense of heaviness in the shoulder and back, upper extremity weakness, cutaneous hypaesthesia in limbs, holding weakness in hands, and sometimes objects held may fall to the ground unconsciously. In other patients it may be accompanied by lower extremity weakness, an unsteady gait and numb feet. They may feel like stepping on cotton when walking.

3. TAPING METHOD FIG. AND TECHNIQUE DESCRIPTION

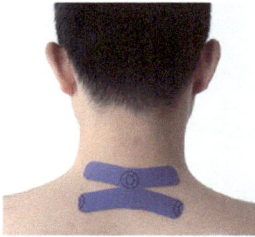

THE FIRST KINTAPE
First apply the middle of the kintape onto the sore spot loosely; stretch the four corners gently to apply it.

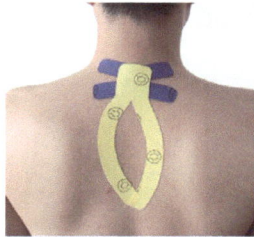

THE SECOND KINTAPE
First apply the junction of the Y-type kintape onto the sore spot loosely. Apply the two branches toward the dorsal vertebrae along the rhomboid muscle.

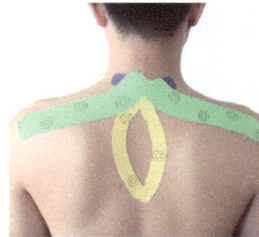

THE THIRD & FOURTH KINTAPES
Apply the I-type kintape toward the neck along the aching muscles of the shoulder in an inward manner.

First: For the X kintape, lower the head forward. Apply the X kintape center onto the sore spot behind the cervical vertebra, making it loose in the middle, and stretching the four sides of the X along the muscle in four directions. Apply the four corners loosely.

Technique: Lift the skin, open the subcutaneous fascia space, and relieve pain at the same time.

Second:	For the Y kintape, keep the same posture. First, apply the connection point of the Y kintape in the middle of the Y with upper edge as high as or higher than that of the X kintape. Next, apply the lower edge arc toward the dorsal vertebrae while stretching onto the edge of the rhomboid muscle and joint in the dorsal vertebrae.
Technique:	Lift the skin space to be applied. Meanwhile, import the dorsal vertebrae lymph into the cervical vertebra to eliminate inflammation. Improve and rebuild fascia channels and relax the rhomboid muscle. Note: apply two branches onto the connection line of the rhomboid muscle and trapezius.

Third/Fourth:	The third and fourth kintapes are I-type ones. Apply the kintape from the shoulders to the neck while stretching onto stiff muscles, and ending the tape at the two bevel sides of the neck roots.
Technique:	Work on muscle and flow guidance simultaneously to relax tense muscles and increase the sluggish blood volume of damaged muscles.

4. REACTIONS AFTER APPLYING

Patients may have the sensation of being stretched when they are applied with kintape. Generally, the muscles will become relaxed after one night. If the neck had an abnormal sound before, the symptom may be relieved after applying.

III. SCAPULOHUMERAL PERIARTHRITIS (PERIARTHRITIS OF SHOULDER)

1. CAUSE OF DISEASE
a. Trauma and movement reduction of shoulder joints;
b. Retrogressive change of scapulohumeral soft tissue;
c. Long-term strain of scapulohumeral ligament, tendon, etc.

2. SYMPTOMS
a. Pain in shoulders: mild in day and severe in night, usually awake due to pain after midnight, cannot lie on the affected side;
b. Patients suffering pains caused by catching a cold are particularly sensitive to changing climates;
c. Pressing pain;
d. Shoulder movements are limited; limited shoulder functions in the case of movements including abduction, upward raising, external rotation, internal rotation, etc. In the later period, some patients have muscle atrophy in their shoulders;
e. Shoulders are sensitive to the chill and wind.

3. TAPING METHOD FIG. AND TECHNIQUE DECOMPOSITION:

First: The claw kintape. Based on the position of the sore spot, apply the connection point onto the joint of the forearm and chest (near the lymph), or apply onto the back (near the lymph). Four claw branches wrap the shoulder fanwise. If the sore spot is in the acromion, the taping method is as shown in Fig.

Technique: The claw flow guidance, with simultaneous acupuncture point effect. Import the blood into the sore spot and lift the subcutaneous space of the sore spot. In case of acromion, import the inflammation into the lymph (when it is ascertained to be a non-bacterial inflammation) to accelerate inflammation elimination.

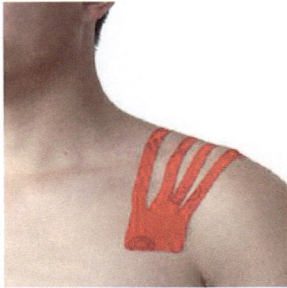

THE FIRST KINTAPE
First apply the claw joint onto the sore spot and the wrap the shoulder fanwise. (The sore spot is the same anywhere)

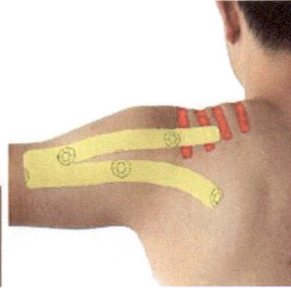

THE SECOND KINTAPE
First apply the Y-type kintape onto musculus triceps brachii in an inward manner (relaxed) with the two branches directing to the shoulder and the back respectively.

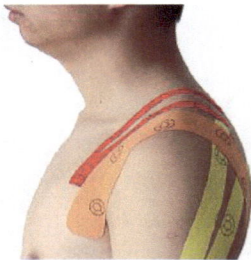

THE THIRD KINTAPE
Apply the I-type kintape onto the front axilla lymph gland from the rear axilla lymph gland through the shoulder.

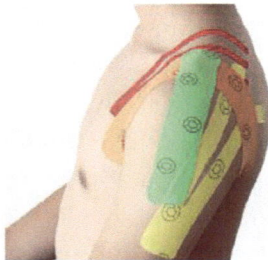

THE FOURTH KINTAPE
Apply the I-type kintape downward onto the edges of the deltoid muscle from the Jianjing acupoint.

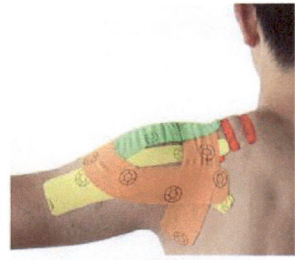

THE FIFTH KINTAPE
Wrap the deltoid muscle with the I-type kintape toward the two sides from the apex of the deltoid muscle.

Second: The Y-type kintape. Raise the arm flat and bend forward to expose musculus triceps brachii. Stretch and apply the kintape from the elbow to the shoulder, then bifurcate in the arm root. Apply two branches of Y-type kintape toward the small intestine meridian and upper edge of the trapezius while stretching.

Technique: Break through meridians and relax the musculus triceps brachii and trapezius connecting to the arm.

Note: if the arm can rotate forward but cannot rotate backward, apply the kintape onto the musculus biceps brachii in the same method. That is, switch to the front or add another kintape in front.

| Third: | The I-type kintape. First apply it onto the rear axilla, then stretch it forward to wrap the acromion and apply it onto the front axilla to form fascia guidance and strength support. |
| Technique: | Import the rear axilla lymph and connect to the front axilla lymph to enhance muscular strength in the shoulder. |

| Fourth: | The I-type kintape. Apply it from the Jianjing acupoint in the shoulder, and then stretch the kintape downward in the middle through the acromion until reaching the lower edge of the deltoid muscle to strengthen the deltoid muscle. |
| Technique: | Form physical lift of the shoulder and accelerate the blood backflow simultaneously. |

| Fifth: | The I-type kintape. Apply the kintape along the middle part from the deltoid muscle. Stretch the two ends upward along the edge arc of the deltoid muscle to wrap the deltoid muscle. |
| Technique: | Strength support. |

4. REACTIONS AFTER APPLYING

Relief in symptoms, including difficulty in raising upward as well as forward and backward rotation. In the case of the deep pain, it will be relieved significantly when pressed with the hands after applying.

IV. LOWER BACK PAIN

1. CAUSE OF DISEASE

a. Keeping the same posture for a long time, causing back rigidity in the relevant muscle group;
b. Incorrect posture when working at a table causes laceration of the muscle;
c. Usual repetition of the same action causes muscle fatigue damage.

2. SYMPTOMS

a. Small muscle stiffness;
b. Muscular soreness;
c. Arm weakness;
d. Obvious pain when pressing with hands.

3. TAPING METHOD FIG. AND TECHNIQUE DESCRIPTION

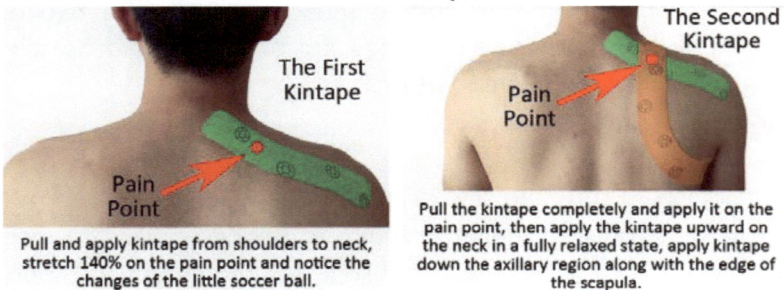

The First Kintape

Pain Point

Pull and apply kintape from shoulders to neck, stretch 140% on the pain point and notice the changes of the little soccer ball.

The Second Kintape

Pain Point

Pull the kintape completely and apply it on the pain point, then apply the kintape upward on the neck in a fully relaxed state, apply kintape down the axillary region along with the edge of the scapula.

First: Pull and apply the kintape from the shoulders to the neck, and stretch it a little more on the pain point and end on the neck.

Technique: Relax tense shoulder muscles to relieve the feeling of tearing pain, and lift the subcutaneous space at the pain point.

Second: Stretch and apply the kintape on the pain point, then stretch and apply the kintape upward on the neck in a fully relaxed state. Lastly, stretch and apply and twine the kintape down the axillary region along with the scapula.

Technique: Wrap the pain point and lift the subcutaneous space, and guide into the lymph of the axillary region, straighten out the fascia tissue along with the scapula. Meanwhile, properly intensify the back muscles to increase lifting capacity.

4. REACTIONS AFTER APPLYING

Pain reduces 50% immediately after applying the kintape. When exerting force on the original pain point, only deep pain is felt.

5. NOTE

This section is called lower back pain but the Fig. shows the meeting part of the scapula muscle and trapezius muscle. The integrated program of the aforesaid kintapes can be adopted within the scope of the latissimus dorsi muscle extended from the pain point. Only adjust the part of the kintape according to different parts of the pain point.

V. STRAIN OF LUMBAR MUSCLES

1. CAUSE OF DISEASE
   a. Chronic injury of supraspinal and interspinous ligaments, excessive waist movement and overload;
   b. Air temperature is too low or humidity is too great;
   c. Retrogressive pelvospondylitis of lumbar vertebra;
   d. Muscle, fascia and ligament damage.

2. SYMPTOMS
   a. The lower waist feels acid pain and weakness when bending over, or the waist feels breakage;
   b. With pain referred towards the bottom; without kinaesthesia disturbance;
   c. There are pressing pains for the superficial tissue among lumbar vertebra 4, 5 or waist 5, sacrum 1 the upper spinous process and spinous process.

3. TAPING METHOD FIG. AND TECHNIQUE DESCRIPTION

The First & Second Kintapes

The Third Kintape

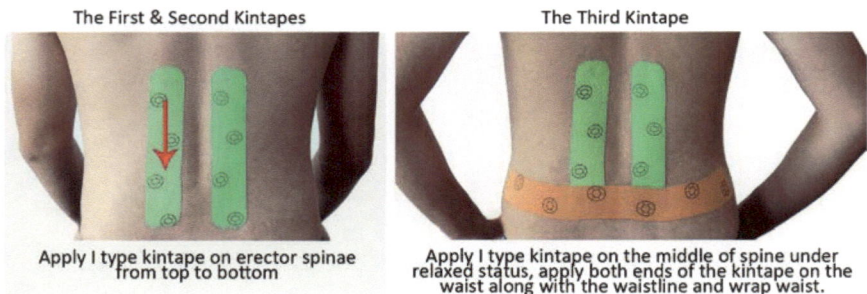

Apply I type kintape on erector spinae from top to bottom

Apply I type kintape on the middle of spine under relaxed status, apply both ends of the kintape on the waist along with the waistline and wrap waist.

First/Second: With the first and second kintapes, stretch and apply them on the erector spinae from top to bottom (located in upheaval part on both sides of the lumbar vertebra, i.e., about 5 cm on the left and right sides of the lumbar vertebra).

Technique: Intensify the strength of the erector spinae of the waist, meanwhile accelerating the blood backflow of the waist.

Third:	Apply the kintape on the pit of the lumbar vertebra, and stretch and apply the kintape toward both sides along the waistline.
Note:	a. The two vertical-I type shall not exceed the Zhishi acupoint (lumbar eye).
	b. There are certain method requirements for horizontal-I type: the middle point of the lumbar vertebra shall be in a fully relaxed state. Then, gently pull about one fingerbreadth wide and press it, then pull completely to the aforesaid kintapes, and stretch and apply the kintape immediately over the meeting part of the aforesaid kintapes.
Technique:	Open the subcutaneous space of the middle part and lift the skin, wrap the zhishi acupoint and lift the space to intensify waist strength.

4. REACTIONS AFTER APPLYING

If the strain of lumbar muscles is at the stage of attack/spasm, the strain is reduced by nearly 30% immediately after applying the kintape. After exercise, a patient with good somatosensory can remove discomfort immediately.

VI. PROTRUSION OF LUMBAR INTERVERTEBRAL DISC

1. CAUSE OF DISEASE

Protrusion of the lumbar intervertebral disc is also called herniation of the nucleus pulposus of the lumbar vertebra, or rupture of the fibrous rings of the lumbar vertebra. Causes are complicated; some causes of the disease are not clearly known.

a. Metamorphosis of the lumbar vertebra and intervertebral discs themselves and trauma;
b. Retrogressive change of lumbar intervertebral disc;
c. Suddenly bearing load; trauma of waist; abdominal pressure increase; external cold-dampness; pregnancy.

2. SYMPTOMS

a. Pain in back and loin in the earlier stage; pain is mainly in the lower waist or lumbosacral portion;
b. Lower limbs on one side have radiating pain, while areas dominated by nerves are still numb and feel cold;
c. Scoliosis malformation, anteflexion, and rear protraction activities of the spine are limited, with the limited lateral bending often on one side;
d. Pressing pain of the waist with radiating pain and circumscribed pressing pain for the side spinous process in the part of the protrusion of the intervertebral disc, with pain radiating towards the shank or foot;
e. Muscle atrophy for a long time may cause ischemia and anoxia degeneration of nerve roots, and result in numbness of the nerves and paralysis of the muscles.

3. TAPING METHOD FIG. AND TECHNIQUE DESCRIPTION

The First Kintape

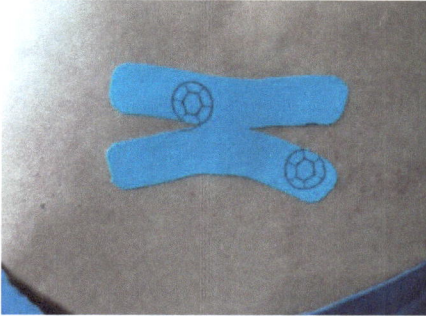

Apply the middle of the X kintape on the pain point of the lumbar vertebra, and pull the four branches towards periphery and apply them

The Second Kintape

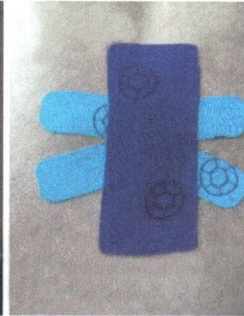

Pull and apply the middle part of kintape. Apply both ends in a relaxed state

The Third & Fourth Kintape

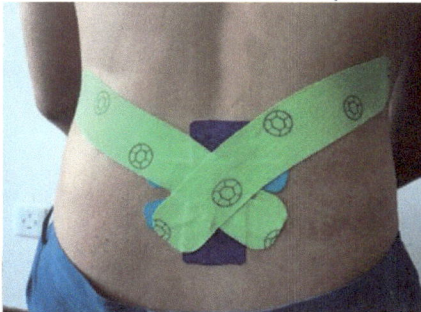

Pull and apply kintape on lumbar vertebra, obliquely apply kintape on waist

The Fifth Kintape

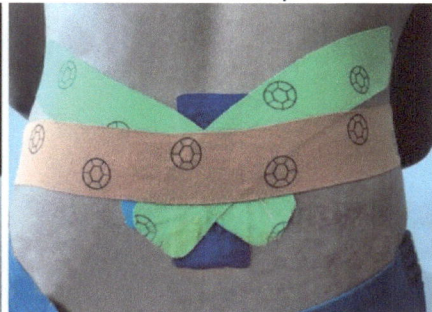

Pull gently and apply the middle of kintape on lumbar vertebra, and then apply kintape on waist along thewaistline.

First: For the X kintape, apply the middle of the kintape on the pain point in a fully relaxed state and gently stretch and apply the four corners of the kintape. The direction of the X kintape shall be perpendicular to the lumbar vertebra.

Technique: The pain point is often the fascia adhesion, open the subcutaneous space with the X kintape.

Second: The I-type kintape is perpendicular to the first kintape, stretch the middle part of the kintape completely and apply it on the X kintape, with both ends in a fully relaxed state.

Technique: Further lift the middle part and wrap the pain point.

Third/Fourth: Stretch them on the pain point, then obliquely apply downward with one side under a fully relaxed state and do not exceed the waistline. Gently stretch and apply up the longer side, along the direction of the latissimus dorsi muscle.

Technique: Flow guidance to increase blood supply of the lumbar vertebra, meanwhile making the nucleus of the vertebra go back to the original place by oppression. It has the role of properly increasing the strength support in the waist.

Fifth: Stretch gently and apply the middle of the kintape on the middle of the lumbar vertebra, then gently stretch and apply both ends of the kintape toward both sides, and twine the waistline.

Technique: provide the waist with strength support, meanwhile transferring the strength bearing of the lumbar vertebra point.

4. REACTIONS AFTER APPLYING

On the acute stage, users will be able to relax more after applying the kintapes. Some patients who could not walk with the injury can now do some exercise. If it is not on the acute stage, there is no obvious feeling; no effects are even felt. Using the kintapes on the acute stages to relieve pain (multiple applications will be needed) can delay the time of onset again.

VII. TENNIS ELBOW (LATERAL EPICONDYLITIS)

1. CAUSE OF DISEASE
a. Hands and wrist are used with repeated force, and feel fatigued;
b. The main cause of pain is myofascitis of muscle insertion, which causes strangulation of the neurovascular bundle of the lateral epicondyle insertion.

2. SYMPTOM
a. The outer upper part of the elbow joint has activity pain, and the pain can sometimes radiate upward and downward;
b. It feels that the hands cannot be used with force to grasp objects, and the bend, stretch, and rotation actions of the elbow and wrist can make the pain even worse;
c. There is a regional pressure point on the lateral epicondyle of the humerus, this pressing pain can sometimes diffuse downward. There can also be mild pressing pains and activity pains even on the extensor tendon.

3. TAPING METHOD FIG. AND TECHNIQUE DESCRIPTION

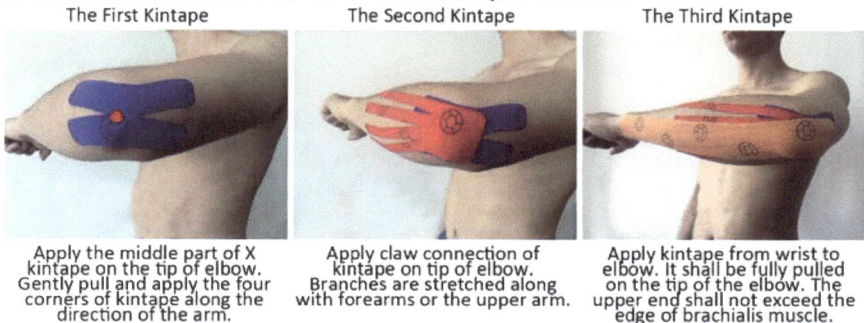

The First Kintape	The Second Kintape	The Third Kintape
Apply the middle part of X kintape on the tip of elbow. Gently pull and apply the four corners of kintape along the direction of the arm.	Apply claw connection of kintape on tip of elbow. Branches are stretched along with forearms or the upper arm.	Apply kintape from wrist to elbow. It shall be fully pulled on the tip of the elbow. The upper end shall not exceed the edge of brachialis muscle.

First: Apply the connection point of the X kintape on the pain point, and then apply the stretched 4 branches towards the upper arm and forearms.

Technique: The main pain points of tennis elbow are in the sutura of the humerus. The X kintape can effectively increase the space under the skin, to provide a strangulated neurovascular bundle with more space.

Second:	Apply the claw kintape pain point first, and then determine the direction of the 4 branches of the claw kintape according to the radiance direction of pain. If pain is radiating upward, apply 4 branches upward. If pain is radiating downward, apply 4 stretched branches downward. An example shown in the Fig. is pain radiating downward.
Technique:	Increase the blood supply of the pain point by blood import, and cover the radiating pain to increase the touch nerve input.
Third:	Apply the I type kintape from the edge of the palm and stretch it while applying the kintape upward. Stretch slightly on the tip of the elbow, and relax to apply the kintape outside of the elbow tip. The whole kintape shall not exceed the edge of the brachialis muscle.
Technique:	Form the channel of blood flow and nerves, relax the muscular tension caused by neuropathic pain, and relax the oppressed nerve bundle. This trend is reverse flow guidance, which can increase the blood stock in muscle groups and deep muscles.

4. REACTIONS AFTER APPLYING

There is no immediate reaction after applying, as the symptoms of tennis elbow are difficult to handle because of the cause of disease in the deepest place. Many repeated uses can reduce pain. For pain caused by occupation (such as carpenters or assembly-line workers), it is more difficult to achieve a satisfying effect. Even though the aforesaid method is used repeatedly many times, it can only release pain. Add other products for relaxing muscles or far IR products, such as vitality cream or nano gold four-way Spandex, as an integrated program.

VIII. GOLFER ELBOW

1. CAUSE OF DISEASE
a. Similar to pathogenesis of tennis elbow, accumulation injury of the medial epicondyle of the humerus with the origin of forearm flexor because of repeated traction;
b. Over fatigue of the original part of the pronatoflexor muscle tendon;
c. Inflammation of muscle tendon within the inner side of the elbow;
d. The soft tissue of the elbow has suffered repeated slight trauma;
e. Using wrist or forearm muscles too much.

2. SYMPTOMS
a. There is pressing pain on joints nearby within the inner side of the elbow;
b. There may be swelling, heat, and pain within the inner side of the elbow;
c. When the finger, wrist, or forearm use force, the inner side of the elbow or forearm will feel pain and a strength deficiency.

3. TAPING METHOD FIG. AND TECHNIQUE DESCRIPTION

The First Kintape	The Second Kintape	The Third Kintape

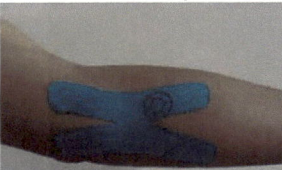

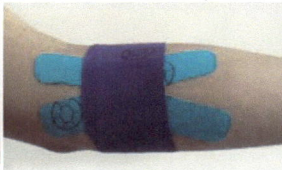

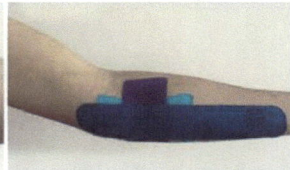

Apply the middle part of kintape at the sore spot. Gently pull and apply the four corners of kintape along with the direction of arm.	The middle part of kintape is stretched and both ends of kintape are relaxed, and Perpendicular to the first kintape	Apply kintape from wrist to elbow and stretch it gently on pain point

First: Apply X kintape on pain point in a relaxed state and stretch the periphery to apply (or stretch the middle and keep the periphery in a relaxed state to apply). Its direction is along the direction of the arm.

Technique: Open the subcutaneous space of pain points to relieve pain.

Second:	For the little I type: apply the kintape on the pain point, perpendicular to the first kintape, with the middle stretched open fully and both sides relaxed.
Technique:	Wrap the pain point and increase the subcutaneous space, meanwhile intensifying the strength of the muscle near the pain point.
Third:	For the I type: apply the kintape in the direction of wrist to elbow, stretching it gently on the pain point. The whole kintape shall not past the elbow, or only pass the tip of the elbow slightly. Note: when using hands to grasp heavy objects, if the thumb has no strength, apply the kintape to the extensor muscle group of the thumb. If the little finger has no strength, apply the kintape to the extensor muscle group of the little finger.
Technique:	Relax the thumb's or little finger's muscle group, give them enough rest, and make blood form an accumulation pressure in the muscle group.

4. REACTIONS AFTER APPLYING

Pressing pain obviously reduces or disappears after applying the kintape, and the tension state of the muscle disappears.

IX. WRIST

1. CAUSE OF DISEASE
    a. Sequela of wrist sprain;
    b. Injury by collision, dotted pain;
    c. Accumulated damage caused by working with the hands; keeping the same posture for a long time;
    d. Damage or inflammation of the muscle tendon.

2. SYMPTOMS
    a. There is pressing pain on the front side or the reverse side of the wrist;
    b. There is an ache in twisting or bending the wrist;
    c. When the wrist is bearing force, there will be a deep ache in the wrist along with a loss of strength;
    d. The exercise scope of the wrist is limited;
    e. When the wrist is lifting heavy objects, it will lose strength and there will be a grip strength deficiency.

3. TAPING METHOD FIG. AND TECHNIQUE DESCRIPTION

The First Kintape

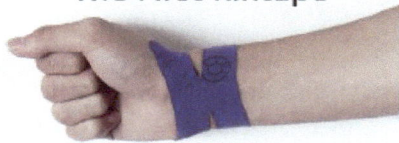

Apply the middle part of kintape on the
center of wrist (pain face), gently pull
and apply four branches.

The Second Kintape

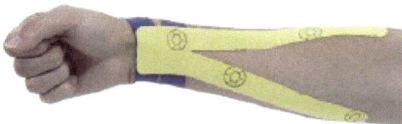

Apply Y type kintape on pain point of
wrist, and apply branches along the
muscle group of thumb and little finger.

The Third Kintape

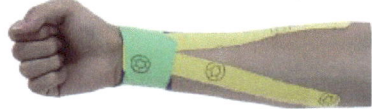

Apply one end of kintape on pain point,
and apply the circle along the wrist

First:	In a relaxed state, apply the middle part of the X kintape on the pain point of the wrist, then apply the kintape on the palm for relieving its pain. Next, apply the kintape on the reverse side of the wrist to relieve its pain. Gently stretch the 4 branches of the release paper while applying the kintape. The elastic force direction of the X kintape should be perpendicular to the direction of the arm.
Technique:	Open the subcutaneous space of the pain point. To prevent blocking the blood channel of the wrist and causing sore and swollen hands, the 4 branches cannot be pulled too far open

Second:	Apply the connection point of the Y-type kintape on the center point of the previous X kintape, then gently stretch the 2 branches while applying them along the muscle groups of the thumb and little finger. The lengths of the branches shall not pass the elbow joint.
Technique:	Relax the forearm muscle to supply blood to the damaged point and promote blood circulation.

Third:	Apply one end of the I type kintape on the pain point, then wrap the wrist clockwise, stretched it while applying the kintape. Note: 1. Only pull the paper, do not pull the fabric. 2. The length of the kintape shall not be too long, and one circle is best.
Technique:	Form fascia recombination on the wrist and ring flow guidance, and make the final import point the pain point of the wrist.

4. REACTIONS AFTER APPLYING

Pressing pain disappears or becomes slight; when using force to press hands perpendicularly, the wrist feels relaxed and the same as the normal wrist.

X. KNEE

1. HANDLING TO THIS SET
   a. Meniscus injury;
   b. Gonarthromeningitis;
   c. Injuries of medial and lateral collateral ligament;
   d. Rectus femoris injury.

2. SYMPTOMS
   a. Pain and weakness;
   b. Cannot bear weight;
   c. Feeling of friction within the knee;
   d. Difficulty walking up and down stairs;
   e. Difficulty squatting, function limited;
   f. Pain when rotating the knee to the inner or outer side;
   g. Swelling and pain in the local part, and flexion and extension of the knee-joint are limited.

3. TAPING METHOD FIG. AND TECHNIQUE DESCRIPTION

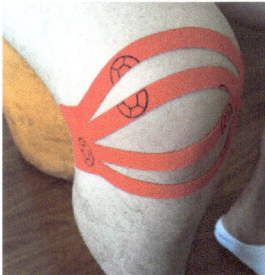

THE FIRST KINTAPE
Apply the claw kintape around the peak of the knee, with the branches stretched around it. Make sure to pull the paper, not the fabric.

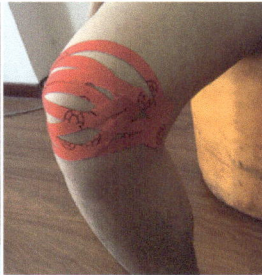

THE SECOND KINTAPE
Use the same method to apply a kintape on the other side of knee. The branches should form diamond crossing wrap on the peak of knee.

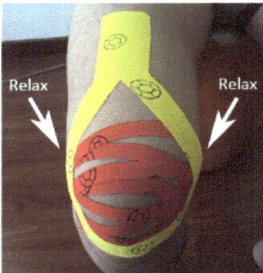

THE THIRD KINTAPE
Apply kintape from the thigh over the knee, to meet on the bottom of the kneecap.

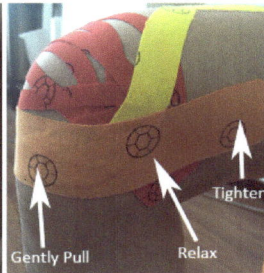

THE FOURTH KINTAPE
Apply the middle of the kintape to the kneecap, then along the sides of the knee and thigh. The tape should be relaxed when applied over the other tapes.

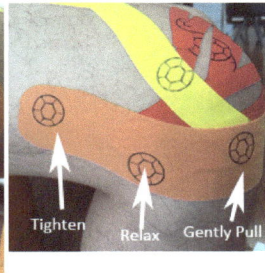

Posture:	Sitting posture of patient during application is with the knee bent at a right angle between thigh and shank.
First/Second:	For the claw kintapes: the starting points are the middle connecting line between the left and right popliteal space of the knee and the peak of the knee respectively. Apply these kintapes on the middle of this connecting line. The elastic direction of the kintape should be the same as the direction of this connecting line. The starting point of the kintape should be applied in a related state and cannot be stretched. The upper two branches of each claw are arched to wrap above the peak of the knee, while the lower two branches of each claw are arched to wrap below the peak of the knee, which forms a rhombic cross on the knee.
Note:	a. When applying the branches of the claw kintapes, do not pull the fabrics, only pull the paper to avoid skin damage and itching. b. The length of the branch of the claw kintape may sometimes exceed the range of the knee, extending to the side edge of the leg (outside of range of the knee's peak). If this happens, the extra length must be cut to prevent leg acidity.
Technique:	Form blood circulation on the peak of the knee and lead to the popliteal space lymph gland.
Third:	For the long-Y type: the connection point of this kintape (like the I type) shall be little longer. Tear off the backing paper about 5 cm from the head of the kintape, then tear off the paper on the connection point and branch point and apply the aforesaid head of the kintape about 5 cm from the face of the thigh (rectus femoris) in a relaxed state; do not stretch here (to prevent skin damage). Then stretch the kintape slowly to the peak of the knee while applying it. Stop stretching the kintape and apply in a relaxed state from the peak of the knee till it reaches the end of the rectus

femoris (do not exceed the rectus femoris). Pull the two branches of the Y type kintape respectively. On the slant side of the face of the knee (like the Fig. above), the stretched degree shall not exceed 120% (to prevent acidity and swelling in the face of the thigh). The meeting part between it and the aforesaid claw kintape over the side shall be in a relaxed state. Then, gently pull the two branches to bend them to the kneecap. The two branches will meet each other in the middle of the face of the kneecap (not downward or upward).

Technique: Rectus femoris segment (the face of the thigh) is to intensify the rectus femoris and accelerate the blood backflow, increasing oxygen content of blood, to effectively increase leg lift strength. The 120% stretch turning to the side is to avoid cutting off the quadriceps and causing insufficient blood supply. The meeting part between it and the aforesaid claw kintape in a relaxed state is to ensure that the flow guidance channel of the claw kintape is not cut off, and to avoid the kintape turning up when the patient is standing up. Gently stretch the kintape when turning to the kneecap to support the kneecap and to avoid the invasion of cold air to protect the kneecap.

Fourth: For the long-I type: tear off the paper from the middle of the kintape. Apply the middle on the kneecap and use the hands to press it tight to the knee. Then, without moving, apply a length of kintape about one fingerbreadth wide with the stretch rate of 140%. Next. apply the kintape firmly, in a fully relaxed state, passing the sides of the knee (where the other kintapes meet). Once the kintape exceeds the meeting part, stretch the kintape nearly 160% to the root of the thigh and apply it on collateral ligaments. Apply the end of the kintape about 5 cm from the side of the thigh in a fully relaxed state and use the same method on the left and right halves of the I-type kintape.

Technique: Keep the kneecap in fully relaxed state. Each one fingerbreadth wide section bearing the force of both sides to lift the kneecap and accelerate blood circulation. The relaxed application where the other kintapes meet is to preserve the circulation channels established by the aforesaid two kintapes. Stretching over the channel and applying upward are to intensify internal and external collateral ligaments respectively, to increase the shuffling capacity of the patient. The integration of these kintapes is to lift the knee and effectively increase the force of the knee.

4. REACTIONS AFTER APPLYING

a. Weakness of legs gets immediate relief, and the ease of walking up and down stairs and the force of the legs increases.

b. For patients with severe cold air, there may be bubble exudations on the skin and itchiness. They will disappear by adjusting the stretch degree and applying many times.

c. For some patients, there may be heating of the knee.

d. Four hours after applying the kintape, some patients may feel cool knees, like the feeling of a spring breeze blowing, and some patients may feel wet knees when they are in fact dry.

e. Aforesaid symptoms can have obvious relief with continuous use.

XI. SHANK ACID

This taping method is aiming at the acid and swelling of the calf after sports; some are adverse reactions because of gastrocnemius muscle damage, calcaneal tendon damage, and muscular tension.

TAPING METHOD FIG.:

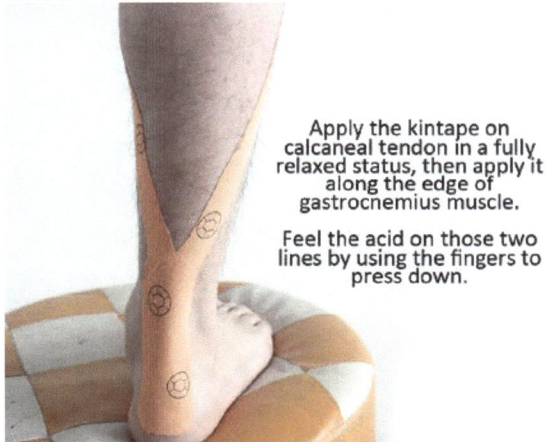

Apply the kintape on calcaneal tendon in a fully relaxed status, then apply it along the edge of gastrocnemius muscle.

Feel the acid on those two lines by using the fingers to press down.

This kintape is Y type. Peel off the release paper on the connection point first. Apply it on the calcaneal tendon in a fully relaxed state. If the calcaneal tendon has damage or if you need to intensify its strength, stretch the middle of the segment, then apply it on the calcaneal tendon. For the two branches of the Y type, pull them along with the edge of the gastrocnemius muscle while applying, stopping at the edge of the soleus muscle. Note: do not apply the kintape on the soleus muscle, or it will become acidic and weak.

The method to find the desired application route: use the thumb and middle finger of your hand to grasp your calf, then use the hand to press down. Those two lines acid you feel on both sides of your shank are the desired two lines; the seam line with muscle connection between the gastrocnemius muscle and soleus muscle.

Technique: Calcaneal tendon intensification, fascia flow guidance, acidic material leads to heel lymph, and relaxes the gastrocnemius muscle.

Reactions: If applied correctly, the acid of the shank gets immediate relief, granting pain relief.

XII. PAIN AND SWELLING OF SHANK

This taping method is aimed at earlier stage symptoms of pain, swelling and varicosity, weakness of the shank, difficulty sleeping because legs are cold or hot at night, acid, and shank numbness in the patient.

TAPING METHOD FIG.:

INSIDE	OUTSIDE

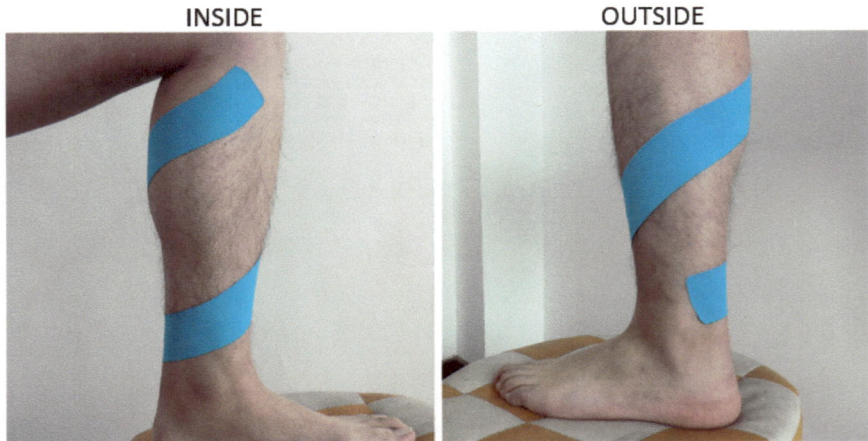

Apply the kintape downward from internal side of knee, under fully relaxed status, rotate and twine the kintape to ankle with tightening at the back of the calf

This kintape is the long-I type: apply the starting point of the kintape on the inner side of the leg, below and near the knee, in a fully relaxed state. Obliquely pull the kintape downward and around while applying, (note, there should be buffering between the starting part and stretching part, or the starting part will form a block-shaped red spot with an itch), around and past the shank, increasing/tightening the stretching degree on the calf, ending on the lymph gland of the ankle.

Technique: Guide the tissue fluid upward. Accelerate the blood backflow and removal of acid materials and the whole fascia recombination. As the oppressive force on the calf increases, the force of the whole shank increases, and the knee nest and lymph gland of the ankle joint connect to rapidly remove inflammation of the legs.

Reactions: Somatosensory will be immediately better. Acid and pain will disappear immediately and exhaustion of the legs decreases. Legs are obviously stronger and the whole leg feels relaxed.

XIII. VARICOSITY

1. CAUSE OF DISEASE
   a. Maintaining the same posture for a long time with rare changes, causing blood to accumulate in the lower limbs;
   b. The venous valve is damaged, causing overly high venous pressure.

2. SYMPTOMS
   a. Telangiectasis and reticular vein dilatation;
   b. Bending and thickening superficial veins can be seen above the skin on the legs when standing, which disappear after lifting the legs or lying down. Often it is accompanied with shank acid bilges and fatiguability;
   c. Shank edema is more apparent after long-term standing or exhaustion, and will fade in the morning. Some itchy skin and skin diseases such as eczema and stasis dermatitis occur;
   d. Local skin becomes red, purple, and even black, losing elasticity and hardening.
   e. Skin ruptures occur and self-healing is difficult;
   f. Ulcers occur repeatedly. It is commonly seen in places near the ankle joint and the lower segment of the shank, which is commonly known as the "old sodden leg".

3. TAPING METHOD FIG. AND TECHNIQUE DESCRIPTION

THE FIRST KINTAPE	THE SECOND KINTAPE

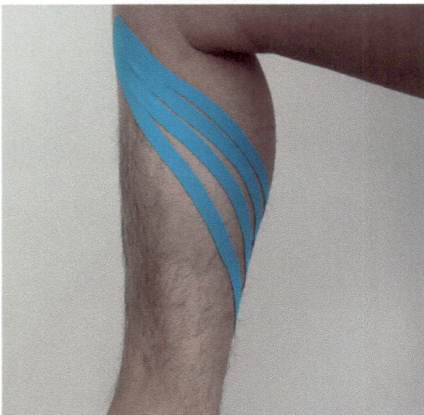

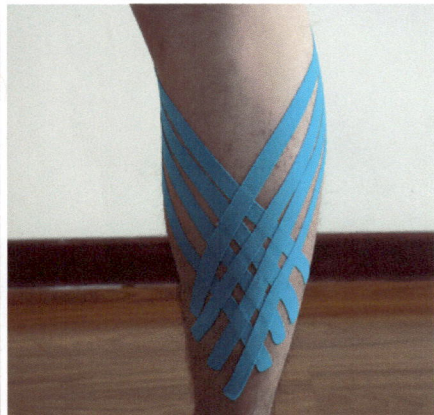

Apply top-down. The claw kintape scatters at the points of varicosity.	Apply the other side top-down. Cross with the former claw kintape at points of varicosity

First:	The first claw kintape has its junction at the upper part near the knee, with the branch stretching down and back to the lower part, stretching and fitting with the part of the varicosity from one side of the leg.
Second:	The second claw kintape, similar to the first taping method but from another side of the leg, meets with the first claw and fan-shaped kintape at the part of the varicosity, forming a diamond crossing. Requirements: stretching is required for both while fitting.
Technique:	a. Two claw kintapes will accelerate the blood circulation and soften hard blocks. b. Divert fluids upward, leading the accumulated blood back to the cardiac. c. Strengthen the blood backflow capability of the legs.

4. REACTIONS AFTER APPLYING

Stretch is required while applying. If it is of slight varicosity, where the branches are the points of varicosity will disappear. If it is severe varicosity, after a time the rigid body surface skin will soften and gradually change color.

Note:	This technical solution is only for relieving the symptoms of varicosity and cannot cure varicosity. With multiple applications, however, it will improve.

XIV. ANKLE SPRAIN

This taping method is aimed at ankle sprains, including treatment of a swollen ankle and precautions after being sprained.

TAPING METHOD FIG.:

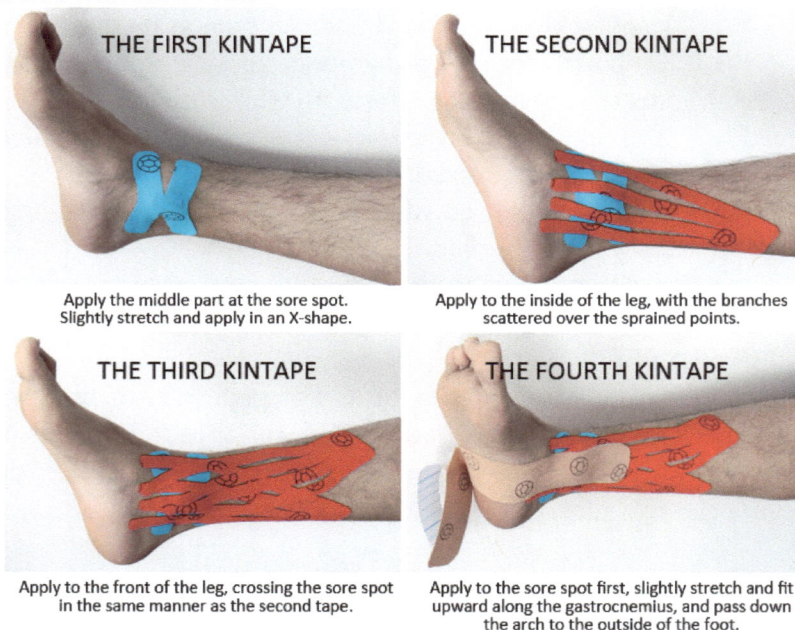

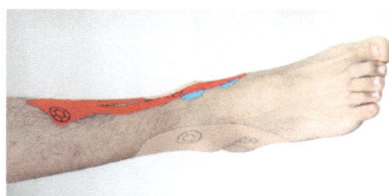

THE FIRST KINTAPE

Apply the middle part at the sore spot. Slightly stretch and apply in an X-shape.

THE SECOND KINTAPE

Apply to the inside of the leg, with the branches scattered over the sprained points.

THE THIRD KINTAPE

Apply to the front of the leg, crossing the sore spot in the same manner as the second tape.

THE FOURTH KINTAPE

Apply to the sore spot first, slightly stretch and fit upward along the gastrocnemius, and pass down the arch to the outside of the foot.

Apply the upper end outside, and then apply on the tibialis anterior top-down.

First: The X kintape is applied first. The central point is loosely applied at the first sore spot with slight stretching and fitting at the four corners (if the sore spot is above the skin, choose the method of stretching from the center with the four corners loosened). Ensure the direction of the X kintape's elasticity is consistent with the blood vessels of the foot.

Technique: Sore spot promotion, open the subcutaneous space, and prepare for flow guidance.

Second/Third: For the second and third kintapes, the two claw kintapes both have junctions at the upper part. Apply the upper end first, then the two claw kintapes at both sides of the shank. The four branches of the claw kintape face downward with the angle towards the first sore spot. It is required to stretch while applying, and the branches from the two claw kintapes should form a crossing at the sore spot over the first X kintape.

Technique: Accelerate blood circulation at the sprain. Fully take advantage of the area at both sides of the shank, conducting upward flow guidance to the inflammation generated by a sprain and the accumulated blood. If it has been swollen, it has the function of apocatastasis.

Fourth: For the long-I type: Cut the appropriate size and tear the release paper near the middle position and pull open/stretch the kintape at the tearing place and apply firmly on the sore spots. Then, apply the two sides in a completely relaxed state. Note: for the upward side, apply down-top, stretching and directly applying on the skin surface. Then, apply down-top and according to the treatment method of muscle relaxation or strengthening, relax the muscle of the tibialis anterior. For the downward side, pass by the arch, and add some strength to the inside of the foot while passing the arch. Apply directly for a segment (to prevent flanging), and then divest all the release paper. Afix the upper end first (on the gastrocnemius), and then apply top-down to strengthen the gastrocnemius.

Technique: The I type taping method of stretching from the center supports the sore spot. Relax the tibialis anterior directly upward (without flow guidance) to prevent injuries to the tibialis anterior due to sprain. Under ordinary circumstances, moreover, eversion ankle sprains will cause failure of exertion of the tibialis anterior. Passing by the arch and slightly tightening up can increase the centripetal force of the arch and reduce vibration. Strengthen the gastrocnemius at the inside to transfer the bearing force of the leg from the tibialis anterior to the gastrocnemius.

NOTE:
a. The above mentioned Fig. is an eversion ankle sprain. If it is an inversion ankle sprain, all taping methods share the same applying order while the applied part shall be adjusted accordingly, for example, transfer the force on the gastrocnemius to the tibialis anterior.
b. The X kintape is determined according to the first sore spot. If the first sore spot is not the point identified in the Fig., all the X kintape, claw kintape and I type will synchronously transfer to the new sore spot.
c. Patients with sprains may have multiple sore spots. Since the foot area is limited, if applying is allowed, all the sore spots can be treated together. But if it is easy to generate conflicts among different functions, it shall be treated fractionally according to the principle of priorities.

REACTIONS AFTER APPLYING:
Treating within 5 minutes after being injured generally keeps the ankle from swelling. After applying the kintape, the pain reduces. Pressing with the hand, the deep layer still has pain but is obviously acceptable. The foot and the ankle can be moved continuously.

XV. FLAT FEET (PLANTAR FASCIITIS)

1. CAUSE OF DISEASE
a. Genetic factor, congenital deformity of metatarsal bones;
b. Foot injury or chronic strain;
c. Intrinsic or extrinsic muscle of the foot is week or paralyzed and has spasms.

2. SYMPTOMS
a. Foot pain or discomfort for long periods of standing or walking;
b. Heel ectropium, flat feet, forefoot abduction, swelling of the nodules of the navicular bone, and pressing pain when standing;
c. For later development, flat feet become spasmodic and can cause osteoarthritis complications.

3. TAPING METHOD FIG.

THE FIRST KINTAPE

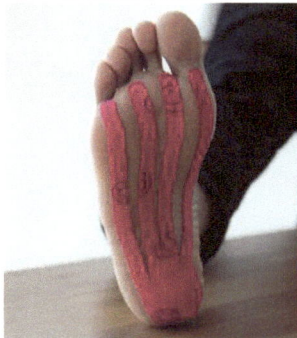

THE SECOND KINTAPE

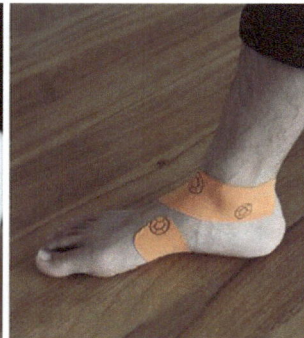

Apply from the heel to the toe

Apply inside the instep. Tighten up while passing the arch, then apply and fit along the ankle

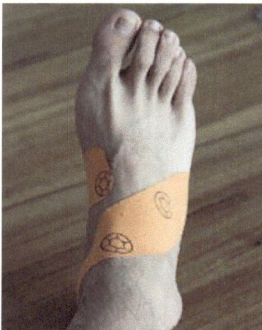

Finished: Above

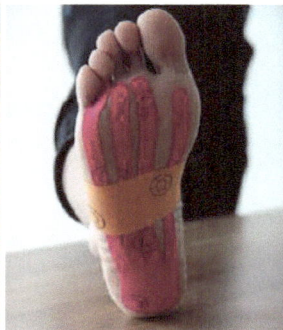

Finished: Below

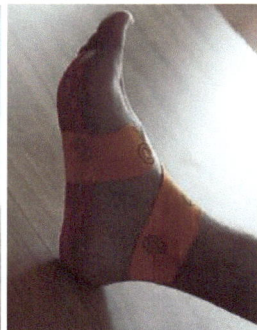

Finished: Side

First:	Apply the claw tape at the heel and the four branches are opened up evenly and toward the toes.
Technique:	Conduct the flow guidance to the fascia plantaris to rapidly remove the acidity.
Second:	Apply the I type from the inside part of the foot edge, slightly stretch the tape and pass by the arch (slightly open up at the arch) and fit in a circular form toward the instep and then surround to the ankle, forming spiral flow guidance support.
Technique:	Promote foot circulation; the lymph of the ankle circulates at the whole foot; under the foot, directly use the physical correction method to promote the instep.

4. REACTIONS AFTER APPLYING

Foot aches and soreness can be removed immediately. Arch feels relaxed. This taping method can also be used for soreness, pain, and swelling of the foot caused by mountain climbing, running, etc.

ABOUT THE AUTHOR

Mr. Han Shibing is the founder and president of DL (Changzhou DL Medical & Health Equipment Co., Ltd - tapes and bandages manufacturer since 2004, the owner of DL and Kintape brand), and is the inventor of Kintape, products of nano-technology and biotechnology. Specialized in technological research and industrialization, he has also studied textiles, electronics, law, and intellectual property, and has been working to break international monopolies of electronics, medical knowledge, and textiles, specifically in the field of Kintape products. In 2015, after nearly ten years of research and testing, Mr. Han completed the Kintape system, including production, usage, and education.

For information about wholesale discounts, please contact Changzhou DL Medical & Health Equipment Co. Ltd. at sales@dlbandage.com

Changzhou DL Medical & Health Equipment Co. Ltd (DL) is the owner of Kintape brand. All Kintapes and practice support is provided By DL. For further information, please visit the DL Website: www.dlbandage.com

For any academic communication, please email to dl@bandage.cn